Manual of Musculoskeletal Medicine

GRANT COOPER, MD

Fellow, Interventional Spine, Sports,
   and Musculoskeletal Medicine
Departments of Orthopedics and Rehabilitation
   Medicine
Beth Israel Medical Center
New York, New York

JOSEPH E. HERRERA, DO, FAAPMR

Director of Sports Medicine
Interventional Spine and Sports Medicine Division
Department of Rehabilitation Medicine
Mount Sinai School of Medicine
New York, New York

D1561392

Wolters Kluwer | Lippincott Williams & Wilkins
Health

Philadelphia · Baltimore · New York · London
Buenos Aires · Hong Kong · Sydney · Tokyo

Acquisitions Editor: Robert A. Hurley
Managing Editor: Dave Murphy
Project Manager: Rosanne Hallowell
Manufacturing Manager: Benjamin Rivera
Marketing Manager: Sharon Zinner
Art Director: Risa Clow
Cover Designer: Melissa Walter
Production Services: International Typesetting and Composition

Printed in China

Library of Congress Cataloging-in-Publication Data

Cooper, Grant, M.D.
    Manual of musculoskeletal medicine / Grant Cooper, Joseph E. Herrera.
        p. ; cm.
    Includes index.
    ISBN-13: 978-0-7817-7919-7
    ISBN-10: 0-7817-7919-7
    1. Musculoskeletal system—Diseaeses—Handbooks, manuals, etc.   I.
Herrera, Joseph E.   II. Title.
    [DNLM: 1. Musculoskeletal Diseases—diagnosis.   2. Musculoskeletal
Diseases—therapy.   3. Musculoskeletal System—injuries.   4.
Pain—diagnosis.   5. Pain—therapy.   WE 141 C776m 2008]
    RC925.5.C66 2008
    616.7—dc22

                                                        2007049655

Care has been taken to confirm the accuracy of the information presented and to
describe generally accepted practices. However, the authors, editors, and publisher
are not responsible for errors or omissions or for any consequences from application
of the information in this book and make no warranty, expressed or implied, with
respect to the currency, completeness, or accuracy of the contents of the publication.
Application of this information in a particular situation remains the professional
responsibility of the practitioner.

The authors, editors, and publisher have exerted every effort to ensure that drug
selection and dosage set forth in this text are in accordance with current recommendations and practice at the time of publication. However, in view of ongoing
research, changes in government regulations, and the constant flow of information
relating to drug therapy and drug reactions, the reader is urged to check the package
insert for each drug for any change in indications and dosage and for added warn-
ings and precautions. This is particularly important when the recommended agent is
a new or infrequently employed drug.

Some drugs and medical devices presented in this publication have Food and
Drug Administration (FDA) clearance for limited use in restricted research settings.
It is the responsibility of health care providers to ascertain the FDA status of each
drug or device planned for use in their clinical practice.

The publishers have made every effort to trace copyright holders for borrowed
material. If they have inadvertently overlooked any, they will be pleased to make
the necessary arrangements at the first opportunity.

To purchase additional copies of this book, call our customer service department at (800) 638-3030 or fax orders to (301) 223-2320. International customers
should call (301) 223-2300.

Visit Lippincott Williams & Wilkins on the Internet: at LWW.com. Lippincott
Williams & Wilkins customer service representatives are available from 8:30 am
to 6 pm, EST.

10 9 8 7 6 5 4 3 2

To my wife Ana, for giving it all meaning.

—GC

To my wife Sandra, for providing inspiration, support, and encouragement.

—JH

Contents

Preface

Musculoskeletal complaints are among the most common reasons for a patient to visit the doctor. "Back pain" alone is the second most common reason for a patient to visit a primary care physician. Despite the ubiquity of musculoskeletal complaints, there remains a lack of comfort in most physicians faced with these complaints. All too often, patients are managed on nonsteroidal anti-inflammatory drugs (NSAIDs) and pain killers until the pain progresses to the point that they are referred to orthopedists for surgical evaluation. Orthopedists for their part might be less familiar with conservative care algorithms and end up referring to a nonsurgical sports medicine doctor or physiatrist.

This *Manual of Musculoskeletal Medicine* provides a step-by-step practical approach to the diagnosis and aggressive nonsurgical management of the most common musculoskeletal complaints. Each section opens with a diagnosis and treatment algorithm section for common chief complaints (e.g., "shoulder pain," "anterior knee pain"). Broad strokes are used to give the clearest possible picture of the complaint and how it should be approached and managed in a logical stepwise fashion.

Of course, any time a book seeks to review a large amount of material and condense it into the highest-yield and most user-friendly points possible, it runs the risk of oversimplification. Please note that the *Manual of Musculoskeletal Medicine* is not intended to replace more detailed texts. This book provides a structural framework into which the reader can add details and nuances gained from further reading and clinical experience.

Ideally, *Manual of Musculoskeletal Medicine* will give the internist and family practice physician enough information to feel comfortable seeing and initially managing musculoskeletal complaints. With the information provided, the general practitioner should recognize when he or she can provide appropriate care and when it is time to refer to a specialist. Also, the general practitioner can use this book to identify when a musculoskeletal complaint is an emergency situation and when a complaint deserves surgical evaluation.

A physiatrist or other nonsurgical musculoskeletal medicine specialist can use this book to guide diagnosis and treatment approaches. Importantly, too, the nonsurgical specialist should also use this book to help identify when it is appropriate to refer for a surgical consultation.

Finally, an orthopedist or neurosurgeon can use this book to review diagnosis and aggressive nonsurgical management algorithms. Of course, this book will not turn a surgeon into a nonsurgeon. Rather, when a patient presents to a surgeon with "back pain" or is being referred for a possible fusion for a "herniated disc," the surgeon may use this book as a review to make certain that appropriate diagnosis and aggressive nonsurgical care have first been provided before considering the surgical option.

Acknowledgments

Several people made this book possible. Many thanks are due to my co-author, Dr. Joe Herrera. I couldn't ask for a better colleague and friend. Thank you, too, to Lippincott Williams & Wilkins. Our editor, Bob Hurley, has been extremely helpful. His commitment and experience helped bring this project to fruition. Thank you to Eileen Wolfberg, our program coordinator at LWW. Eileen's wit, spirit, and passion were indispensable in putting this book together. Thank you also to Dave Murphy, the managing editor for this book. Dave was responsible for a lot of the heavy lifting to bring this project to fruition, and I am grateful for him.

Thank you to my lovely wife Ana, who, in addition to all of the other things she does, served as the model for the pictures in this book.

It is a privilege also to have the opportunity to say thank you to Dr. Robert Gotlin, Dr. Stuart Kahn, and Dr. Alexander Lee for their continued mentorship through all that I do. Thank you also to my parents for their continued unwavering encouragement and support. And, finally, thank you to Dragomir, Ljubica, Jason, Aaron, Sharon, Robin, John, Emma, Allison, Viktor, Mark, Bob, and Dr. Holstein for always helping, caring, and supporting me every step of the way.

Grant Cooper, MD

First I would like to thank my co-author Dr. Grant Cooper. Without his vision, energy, and patience this book would not be possible. Thanks to Ana for taking the time to model for the photos in this book. I would also like to mention and thank Bob Hurley and Eileen Wolfberg from Lippincott Williams & Wilkins. A special thanks to Dr. Kristjan Ragnarsson, Dr. Robert Gotlin, Dr. Stuart Kahn, and

Dr. Gregory Mulford for their mentorship, which has helped me develop into the physician I am today.

I would like to thank my parents and my sister Sacha, who have given me the love and support to persevere and succeed.

Joseph E. Herrera, DO

Manual of
Musculoskeletal
Medicine

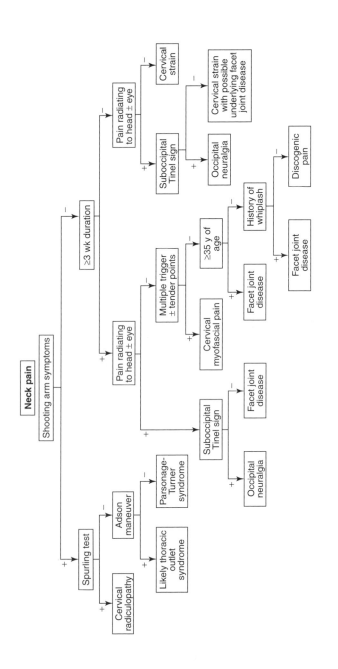

Neck Pain and Shooting Arm Pain

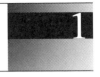

CERVICAL RADICULITIS/RADICULOPATHY

Background

Cervical radiculopathy, as the term is commonly used, is characterized by inflammation and/or compression of the nerve root and/or dorsal root ganglion. The symptoms of cervical radiculopathy typically consist of shooting pain and/or numbness that *radiates* from the neck into the arm and often into the hand. As opposed to other referral pain patterns, which may be diffuse and vague in distribution, radicular symptoms characteristically follow the sclerotome of the involved nerve root. As such, patients can often trace with two or three fingers the distribution of the symptoms as they radiate down the arm (Fig. 1.1). The character of the pain is typically described as "electric," "burning," and/or "sharp." This contrasts with other referral pain patterns, which may be more "dull" and "achy." Cervical radiculopathy also may involve weakness of the muscles supplied by the involved nerve root (Table 1.1).

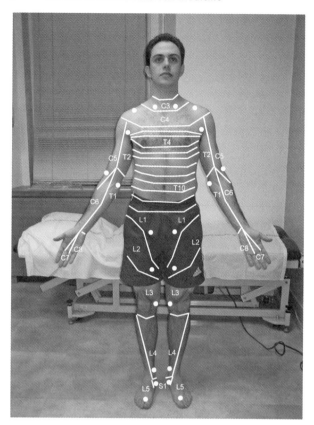

Figure 1.1 Radicular symptoms characteristically follow the sclerotome of the involved nerve root. As such, patients can often trace with two or three fingers the distribution of the symptoms as they radiate down the arm.

In the rare instance that symptoms of a cervical radiculitis/radiculopathy become severe and progressive, or if patients have a sudden change in their bowel or bladder habits (including losing continence), emergent care is necessary and the patient should seek immediate medical attention.

TABLE 1.1
CERVICAL RADICULAR PATTERNS

Root Level	Major Muscle Movements Involved	Reflexes Involved	Decreased Sensation
C5	Weak shoulder abduction; weak elbow flexion	Biceps	Deltoid and lateral anterior elbow crease
C6	Weak elbow flexion; weak wrist extension	Brachioradialis	Dorsal first digit
C7	Elbow extension	Triceps	Dorsal third digit
C8	Finger flexion	None	Dorsal fifth digit
T1	Fifth digit abduction	None	Medial anterior elbow crease

Clinical Presentation

The typical patient presents with several days of neck pain and intermittent shooting, electric pain that radiates in a bandlike fashion down the arm and into the hand. The pain may be positional. Turning the head in the direction of the pain often exacerbates the symptoms. Because of the severity of symptoms, the patient may report having trouble sleeping. The inciting event is typically difficult to identify. However, sometimes, symptoms begin after a traumatic event or exercise, such as after doing a head-stand in certain higher-level yoga positions.

Physical Examination

The most common finding on physical examination is a positive Spurling test. In this test, the patient's head is passively rotated to the side of the pain and extended. Gentle pressure is then placed at the top of the head, directed toward the feet (Fig. 1.2). This maneuver narrows the foramen, putting pressure on the affected nerve root. It is positive when it reproduces the radicular symptoms into the patient's arm. If pain is localized to the neck, the test is not positive. Moving the head to the opposite direction (contralateral rotation and extension) often alleviates symptoms because it takes the pressure off the nerve root.

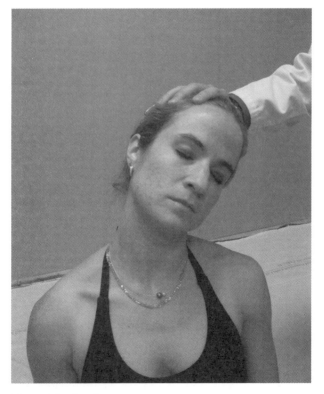

Figure 1.2   Spurling test.

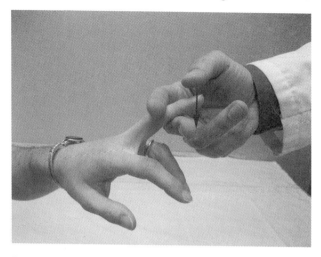

Figure 1.3   Hoffman test.

Sensory deficits may be detected in the distribution of the affected nerve root(s) (Fig. 1.1). Weakness is often subtle but may be detected. Reflexes may also be diminished (Table 1.1).

The Hoffman reflex should be checked (Fig. 1.3). In this test, the middle dorsal finger is "flicked" and if the first or second digit reflexively flexes, the sign is positive and indicates an upper motor neuron problem. The presence of this sign should raise suspicion for a more serious underlying problem such as spinal cord impingement.

Diagnostic Studies

Radiographs should be obtained. These will likely reveal foraminal stenosis, decreased disc height, and spondylosis but will be otherwise normal.

Magnetic resonance imaging (MRI) should be obtained unless symptoms are very mild. MRI may reveal foraminal stenosis from facet hypertrophy (typically in older patients) or a foraminal disc (typically in younger patients).

Electromyelography/nerve conduction studies (EMG/NCS) are not generally needed unless the diagnosis is in doubt or surgery is being contemplated.

Treatment

Treatment generally begins with physical therapy. Physical therapy addresses postural mechanics and gentle range of motion and strengthening exercises. Nonsteroidal anti-inflammatory drugs (NSAIDs) can be used to help quiet the inflammation. Ice (or a bag of frozen peas) can be a very good anti-inflammatory agent for this pathology.

If sleep is affected, a muscle relaxant taken at night may be helpful. Some physicians also suggest offering a nerve-stabilizing medication such as gabapentin (e.g., Neurontin) or pregabalin (e.g., Lyrica), which may help the symptoms.

If symptoms are particularly severe, or the patient wants to be aggressive, an oral steroid taper may be appropriate. One should be cautious, however, when considering an oral steroid taper to ensure it is not used until discitis and other inflammatory as well as malignant causes of symptoms have been ruled out. Oral steroid tapers should not be used for these conditions and may worsen the disease. It may be advisable to get a cervical MRI prior to giving oral steroids.

If the patient does not improve after 3 to 4 weeks of the conservative care just described, a fluoroscopically guided epidural steroid injection may be considered. Epidural steroid injections in the cervical spine are generally well tolerated; devastating adverse events have been reported, however, and so these injections should be respected and only done when more conservative measures have failed. They also may be used sooner if the patient's symptoms are particularly severe and the patient understands the risks. Risks, although rare, include paralysis and death. These injections, like all injections, should only be performed by experienced expert physicians. If the cervical epidural steroid injection is helpful but symptoms persist, a second and possible third injection may be attempted. If the first injection does not help at all, a repeat injection (unless at a different level or from a different approach—transforaminal versus interlaminar) is unlikely to be useful.

If symptoms persist despite aggressive conservative care, including epidural steroid injections, *and* an identifiable pathology is identified on the MRI, surgery should be considered. Progressive symptoms or change in bowel or bladder habits represent a potential surgical emergency and should be evaluated emergently.

CERVICAL STRAIN

Background

The muscles and tendons in the neck can be strained because of chronic, repetitive overuse with poor posture and tension or from an acute injury. The medical definitions in this regard are gray. For the purposes of this book, the diagnosis of "cervical strain" is reserved for an acute condition from a relatively minor trauma (e.g., sleeping "wrong" on the neck one night; twisting too quickly to the side) and the diagnosis of "cervical myofascial pain" is reserved for chronic overuse injuries. The distinction is important because the mechanism of injury is different as is the natural history and treatment. Similarly, neck pain following a major trauma such as a motor vehicle accident (whiplash) is a different category of injury as well.

Clinical Presentation

The typical patient presents complaining of having "slept on the pillow wrong" or looked quickly upward and felt a sharp pain in the neck. For most patients, the pain is not particularly severe, but cervical range of motion is restricted because of the pain. Most patients wait a few days or more before coming to the doctor. When they do come, it is because the pain has not improved. The pain is localized and *does not radiate*. Also, the patient does not complain of numbness, tingling, or weakness. If complaints include radiating electric pain, numbness, tingling, or weakness, suspect a cause other than a simple muscle strain.

Physical Examination

The most common finding on physical examination is focal pain, tenderness, guarding, and decreased neck range of motion. Neurologically (strength, sensation, and reflexes), the patient is intact. If you have the patient lie down and support her neck with your hands (eliminating gravity), you may be able to move her neck passively through a greater range of motion.

Diagnostic Studies

None is generally needed unless looking to exclude other causes of neck pain.

Treatment

Treatment begins with an understanding of the mechanism of injury. Cervical strain is essentially a muscle pull in the neck. Once the neck is injured, the patient stops using it as much and the neck gets stiff. Treatment addresses the inflammation and pain associated with the muscle, and it also looks to increase range of motion gently in the neck.

Ice and/or heat is very good for alternately reducing inflammation and reducing muscle stiffness. Reassurance and education play a prominent role in the treatment of this condition. Patients should be reassured that their condition is common and normal and almost always goes away on its own within a couple of weeks. Patients should be instructed to do *gentle* range of motion exercises. A brief course of physical therapy can be helpful. The therapy can also address any underlying abnormal postural biomechanics or imbalances that may have contributed to suffering the strain. NSAIDs may also be helpful. Occasionally, if symptoms are severe, a muscle relaxant at night may help the patient fall asleep. Restoring a normal sleep cycle is very helpful for recovery.

If symptoms persist for more than 3 weeks despite these treatment measures, an alternative diagnosis should be suspected.

CERVICAL MYOFASCIAL PAIN

Background

This common disorder is a by-product of poor postural mechanics and stress. Patients with this problem often spend a lot of their day hunched over a computer or a stack of papers. Stress also plays a role, leading to further tension being held in the muscles, worsened posture, and decreased tolerance for pain—leading to more tension.

Clinical Presentation

Patients typically report pain over their neck and periscapular areas (around their cervicothoracic paraspinal muscles, rhomboids, and trapezius). The pain does not radiate into their arms. Patients often report that they spend a lot of time sitting at a desk or driving. Usually, the patients do not have an ergonomically optimized work-space, and working tends to aggravate their pain so it is worst toward the end of a long day. Rest often makes the pain better. The pain may have been present for weeks but more usually months or years. The patient finally gets fed up with the pain or comes to see the doctor because the pain has been progressively getting worse.

Physical Examination

Often, the first thing you notice on examination is that the patient has a slumped forward, kyphotic posture. The most common physical examination findings are tight cervicothoracic paraspinal muscles, rhomboids, and trapezius. Tender and/or trigger points are palpable in these areas. Neurologically, the patient is intact.

Diagnostic Testing

No additional testing is needed unless to rule out other potential causes.

Treatment

The cornerstone of treatment is addressing the underlying abnormal postural biomechanics. This begins with ergonomic and postural education. Physical therapy is extremely useful to strengthen the scapular stabilizers, stretch the pectorals, and improve posture. As with all physical therapy, modalities such as heat and ultrasound may make the patient feel better during the therapy session, but for lasting benefit the patient must *do* exercises during therapy and then continue with a home exercise program.

A course of acetaminophen or NSAIDs may also be appropriate in addition to physical therapy.

If trigger points are palpated, trigger point injections can help the patient feel better sooner and have a jump start on the road to recovery (the patient still needs to address the abnormal postural biomechanics or the symptoms will almost surely recur).

CERVICAL FACET JOINT (Z-JOINT) SYNDROME

Background

By far the single most common cause of chronic neck pain (defined as neck pain lasting >3 months) is facet joint pain. The facet joints in the neck are properly termed *zygapophysial joints*, or *Z-joints* for short. In a nod to convention, we use the term *facet joints* in this book. Facet joint pain accounts for as much as 50% of chronic neck pain in patients with a history of whiplash injury. The facet joints facilitate neck flexion, extension, and rotation, and they limit forward displacement and downward displacement. Because of their orientation, the upper and middle cervical facet joints (C3-6) actually contribute more to weightbearing than does the lowest cervical facet joint (C7), which disperses its load onto the laminae. During a high-speed trauma to the neck, the small muscles of the neck are not able to activate in time to protect the facets. The exact etiology of facet joint pain is not known. It is a synovial joint and can suffer the same injuries as any synovial joint (e.g., the knee). In all likelihood, facet joint syndrome originates from a combination of osteoarthritis, repetitive microtrauma, and perhaps a history of macrotrauma.

Anatomic purists will note that because the atlantooccipital joints and C1-C2 both do not reside posterior to the neuraxis, they are not true facet joints.

Clinical Presentation

Patients typically present with a complaint of axial neck pain. The pain is characterized as dull and aching. When the lower facets are involved (C4-7), the pain may radiate into the periscapular area. When the upper facets are involved (C1-3), the pain may radiate from the occiput to the head and eye. Many patients present with predominantly headache with only a mild neck pain. Occasionally, the pain refers down the arm into the hand. As opposed to a cervical radiculitis, the patient generally does not complain of "shooting" "electric" pain or numbness or weakness. In most patients, a history of whiplash injury can be elicited. This injury does not have to happen directly prior to the pain. The injury may be in the distant past, although this may make the relationship less clear.

Physical Examination

No one distinguishing feature on physical examination can make the diagnosis. Neck extension (which loads the facets) may recreate the pain. Neurologically, the patient is intact. Muscles that overlie the facets and facets' referral pain pattern may be tight and tender as a reaction to the underlying facet joint pathology. Some practitioners believe that if patients lie down on their back, the facets can be palpated and that reproduction of the pain signals facet disease.

Diagnostic Testing

Radiographs may show facet arthropathy, but this is not diagnostic of facet joint pain. Likewise, MRI may show facet arthropathy and inflammation, but in the literature this also does not show a good correlation with subsequent relief from injections. Still, obtaining an MRI is important to evaluate the surrounding structures and rule out other pathologies. MRI may also guide where to attempt blocking the facet joints. The only imaging study that shows promise for its ability to diagnose facet joint pain (and this has been in the lumbar spine) is a bone scan with single-photon emission computed tomography (SPECT). This diagnostic approach, however, has not yet replaced the gold standard for diagnosing cervical facet joint pain.

The gold standard for diagnosing facet joint pain is via injection. The facet joints can be injected intra-articularly. Or the medial branch nerves of the dorsal rami that supply the facet joints can be blocked. Because an intra-articular injection may be therapeutic as well as offering diagnostic information, many physicians prefer this method. These injections are generally performed after MRI is obtained. Deciding which facet joints to block is always a tricky equation. Ideally, each facet would be injected individually at one visit. That way, it would be clear *which* facet is the actual cause of pain. In addition, because single blocks of facet joints have about a 24% false-positive rate, double blocks are preferred. In the "real world," however, with real patients and real insurance companies, it is reasonable to inject multiple facets at one time. As a general rule, if the patient has pain in the neck and head, C2-3 and possibly C1-2 and C3-4 should be injected. If the patient has pain in the neck and periscapular region, or pain referred into the arm, then the C4-5, C5-6, and C6-7 should be injected. If the block is positive, the patient should have at least 80% pain relief in at least one area where the pain previously existed.

Treatment

As mentioned earlier, intra-articular injections of the facet joints are often therapeutic as well as diagnostic.

To maximize the chance to improve from these injections, patients should be enrolled in a structured physical therapy program. In fact, sometimes, physical therapy alone provides adequate relief such that the patient does not need to undergo the injections at all.

If the injections provide temporary relief, but the symptoms return, the next step is to perform a radiofrequency rhizotomy of the medial branches supplying the involved facet joints. Prior to performing a radiofrequency rhizotomy, second confirmatory infections should be performed in order to ensure that the facet(s) is the true cause of pain. These infections should be medial branch blocks of the nerves supplyings the joint(s). Once this is done, radiofrequency rhizotomy may be pursued. This procedure essentially burns the medial branches, which cuts the signal from the facet joint to the brain. Without the signal, the patient does not experience the pain. The nerves regenerate over time. They do not always return to cause pain. However, when they do, the procedure may need to be repeated once every 6 months to 2 years. The procedure is done percutaneously under fluoroscopic guidance. When done by an expert experienced physician, the procedure is extremely well tolerated. There are no known adverse reactions to nonfunctioning medial branches.

OCCIPITAL NEURALGIA

Background

Occipital neuralgia is a relatively common and underappreciated cause of headache. The cause is a compression and/or irritation of the third occipital nerve as it passes approximately midway between the mastoid process and suboccipital protuberance. It may also coincide with whiplash injury.

Clinical Presentation

Patients typically complain of a throbbing pain that begins in the suboccipital region and spreads up over the scalp and forehead and into the ipsilateral eye in a bandlike pattern. Patients may use the word *migraine* to describe the pain. Sometimes patients also complain that their neck feels very tight. Of note, this distribution of symptoms is nearly identical to the referral pain pattern of the C2-3 facet joint. The differentiation of the two pathologies is made on physical examination.

Physical Examination

The hallmark sign of occipital neuralgia is reproduction of symptoms by pressing on the occipital nerve, or by performing the Tinel test, approximately midway between the mastoid process and suboccipital protuberance. This physical examination finding distinguishes it from a referral pain pattern of upper cervical (classically C2-3) facet joint, which palpation cannot reproduce in this area.

Diagnostic Testing

Diagnostic studies are generally not indicated.

Treatment

A steroid and anesthetic injection at the point of maximal tenderness can be very effective in treating this condition. Physical therapy that focuses on gentle stretching, range of motion exercises, and postural exercises can also be employed.

If the patient does not respond to the treatment just described, the patient may have upper cervical facet joint pain with an overlying occipital neuralgia. At that point, investigating the facets more closely may be appropriate.

CERVICAL DISCOGENIC PAIN

Background

The cervical discs can be a source of pain; however this is much less common than in the lumbar spine. Patients are typically younger (20s to 40s).

Clinical Presentation

Patients typically complain of severe pain in the axial neck. The pain may refer into the head or scapulae. Because the involved cervical discs are usually C5-6 or C6-7, the pain typically refers in the scapular region. Headache would be a rare presenting symptom. Unless the disc is pressing on a nerve root or the dorsal root ganglion, the patient will not complain of pain shooting into the arm or hand. Rarely, the pain may refer in this distribution, but then the pain will be dull, achy, and poorly localized. The patient will not complain of numbness, weakness, or tingling.

Physical Examination

On physical examination, the patient may have more pain with neck flexion than extension. Range of motion is often restricted because of pain. Neurologically, the patient is intact.

Diagnostic Studies

Radiographs may be helpful. Decreased disc space *may* be seen for the involved disc, but this is not diagnostic. MRI may provide additional information regarding disc desication, degenerative disc disease, inflammatory changes, and the surrounding soft tissues. In the end, however, the gold-standard diagnostic study remains cervical discography. This is an invasive procedure in which contrast dye is injected under pressure into the suspected cervical disc(s) under fluoroscopic guidance. It is more commonly performed in the lumbar spine. In the cervical spine, it should only be performed if a cervical disc replacement or cervical fusion is being considered for suspected discogenic pain. This is a rare incidence and prior to discography, aggressive conservative treatment should be exhausted and other pain generators should be interrogated if suspected.

Treatment

The mainstay of treating presumed cervical discogenic pain is conservative. A soft cervical collar at night can help protect the disc from being uncomfortably torqued at night when the neck muscles relax. However, as with other conditions the collar should not be used during the day because maintaining, and encouraging, full range of motion of the neck is critical to recovery. Ice can be a potent anti-inflammatory agent. NSAIDs are also very appropriate. Often, after obtaining the MRI, a steroid taper is appropriate to help quiet the inflammation in the disc. Physical therapy is also important to help stretch and strengthen the surrounding musculature and also to optimize postural mechanics.

Fluoroscopically guided cervical epidural steroid injection (the interlaminar approach may be best and safest for presumed discogenic pain) may be attempted. This is a relatively dangerous injection in that paralysis and death may rarely result. However, if the patient has not obtained relief from more conservative measures, it may be appropriate.

If all of the preceding measures have failed and the pain is impacting the patient's quality of life, more aggressive measures may be needed. If other pain generators have been ruled out, then cervical discography can confirm the diagnosis of discogenic pain. Once the diagnosis is confirmed, cervical disc replacement and/or cervical fusion are potential further treatments.

CERVICAL MYELOPATHY

Background

Cervical myelopathy is a compressive injury to the spinal cord. Myelopathy actually means "disturbance or disease of the spinal cord." This is a rare occurrence but needs emergent evaluation and treatment when it is found. The underlying pathology is usually a degenerative spine that may include bulging or herniated discs, facet joint hypertrophy, and ligamentous hypertrophy. In addition, some people are genetically predisposed to a myelopathy because of a narrow spinal canal to begin with.

Clinical Presentation

Patients generally do not complain of pain. Instead, they complain of "heaviness" in their arms and/or legs, clumsiness in their hands, and/or unsteady gait. If the symptoms have come on gradually, concomitant foraminal stenosis may be present, in which case the patient may complain of radiating pain and other radicular symptoms. Patients may also complain of loss of bowel or bladder control.

Physical Examination

Depending on the level and degree of involvement, various symptoms may be seen, including hand clumsiness, disturbed gait (e.g., broad based, spastic), weakness, and decreased sensation. Involved reflexes will be hyperreflexic. Clonus may be noted. The Hoffman sign may be present. In this sign, as described previously, the distal interphalangeal joint of the third digit is flicked. If the first or second digit reflexively flexes, the sign is positive and indicates an upper motor neuron problem (Fig. 1.2). The Lhermitte sign, an electrical sensation running down the back and into the legs with neck flexion, may be present and also indicates a myelopathy.

Diagnostic Studies

Cervical myelopathy needs emergent evaluation. Radiographs are routine to get but unlikely to reveal the underlying cause of symptoms. MRI should be obtained. If the patient has a contraindication to MRI, computed tomography (CT) with myelography is a good alternative.

Treatment

A patient with cervical myelopathy should have a surgical consultation. If the symptoms have been progressive, or have developed suddenly, the surgical consultation should be emergent. Surgery is needed to stabilize the spine and prevent further injury. In some cases, depending on the degree of symptoms, progressiveness of the process, and comorbidities, the patient may be managed conservatively. However, a close watch of these patients is required. Unchecked or missed cervical myelopathy can result in permanent catastrophic spinal cord damage.

THORACIC OUTLET SYNDROME

Background

Thoracic outlet syndrome (TOS) is a fairly controversial diagnosis. Various classifications exist to differentiate types of TOS. In general, TOS involves a compressive or other injury to the neurovascular structures in the upper thoracic region at the root of the neck. The scalenes, first rib, cervical rib, pectoralis minor, and other structures have all been implicated. Some have suggested that "true neurogenic TOS" involves clear documentation of nervous abnormalities on EMG/NCS. "True vascular TOS" involves subclavian arterial or venous damage as documented on arteriogram or venogram. "Nonspecific" or "disputed" TOS does not have a clearly documented lesion. Disputed TOS is the most common form.

Clinical Presentation

Patients generally complain of radiating arm pain, numbness, and tingling. The symptoms often sound similar to those of a patient with radiculitis; however, they may be more vague in distribution, including multiple sclerotomes. In addition, autonomic symptoms such as cold hands and blanching are reported.

Physical Examination

Numbness and/or weakness may be found over the distribution of the involved nerves. The most common physical examination test used for evaluating TOS is the Adson maneuver. In this maneuver, the patient is seated and the radial pulse monitored. The patient's head is extended and flexed toward one side and then the other. The patient is instructed to take a deep breath when the head is turned. If the radial pulse diminishes when the head is turned to the affected side, TOS is suspected. However, this test is nonspecific, and many false positives may occur. Another test is to elevate the patient's arm in the abducted and flexed position over the head. If the radial pulse diminishes, or symptoms are reproduced, some physicians believe this outcome suggests TOS.

Diagnostic Studies

Generally, radiographs are all that are needed initially. These films may reveal a cervical rib. MRI may also be useful, although not necessary to begin with, to evaluate for the specific site of impingement. MRI also helps rule out a more serious underlying cause such as a Pancoast tumor if that is suspected. If vascular TOS is suspected, Doppler studies may be helpful. Angiography and venography are invasive but can also be obtained. EMG/NCS can identify true neurogenic TOS if that is suspected.

Treatment

Because postural abnormalities are believed to be responsible for many of the cases, the cornerstone of treatment is physical therapy that focuses on stretching the anterior chest wall and strengthening the scapular retractors (trapezius and rhomboids). Modalities, including ultrasound in particular, can be helpful in helping with physical therapy. Conservative manual manipulation may also be helpful. Surgery is rarely indicated and should be reserved for severe cases where an identifiable lesion is found and conservative care has failed. Complications from surgery in this region include brachial plexus injuries such as injury to the long thoracic nerve.

Note that if the patient is not getting better with good, aggressive, conservative care, it is particularly appropriate with this controversial diagnosis to return to the drawing board and make sure you are not dealing with a different etiology such as a radiculitis that might benefit from a different treatment algorithm.

PARSONAGE-TURNER SYNDROME/ IDIOPATHIC BRACHIAL NEURITIS

Background

Parsonage-Turner syndrome is a relatively uncommon disorder consisting of acute onset shoulder and/or arm pain. It is essentially an idiopathic inflammation of one or more nerves of the brachial plexus. The etiology is unknown, although it has been linked to viral, bacterial, and other immune etiologies, including recent vaccination. Before making the diagnosis, other causes of brachial plexus compression and inflammation (such as a tumor) need to be ruled out.

Clinical Presentation

Patients typically present with acute onset shoulder and/or upper arm pain. Although less common, the forearm and/or hand may also be involved. The pain typically is very severe and described as sharp and/or achy and exacerbated by moving the involved extremity. Moving the neck does not tend to exacerbate the pain. The pain tends to lessen over the course of 1 to 3 weeks, and weakness occurs in the distribution of the involved nerves. Numbness may also be present. Coughing does not aggravate the symptoms.

Physical Examination

During the acute event, patients are in considerable discomfort. They are guarding the involved extremity, often supporting it with the uninvolved side. Examination is limited secondary to pain. The involved muscles are typically tender. As the acute event subsides, atrophy may be noted in the involved muscles. Similarly, weakness, decreased sensation, and diminished reflexes may also be noted in the distribution of the involved nerve(s).

Diagnostic Studies

EMG/NCS should be considered to confirm the diagnosis. However, it may take 1 to 2 weeks before loss of sensory and motor amplitudes is found, and 2 to 3 weeks for needle EMG to show changes.

Radiographs may be obtained. MRI and/or CT myelogram should be obtained to help rule out other etiologies of brachial plexus compression. In addition, if the EMG/NCS are inconclusive, these imaging studies may point toward a radicular etiology.

Treatment

Initial treatment is supportive pain management. Once the pain is under control, the pain medication can be tapered quickly and the patient enrolled in a structured physical therapy program to focus on strengthening and stretching. Steroids are not helpful for this disorder. Most patients make a full recovery within 1 to 2 years. If the patient is not improving or if symptoms continue in a lesser form despite aggressive physical therapy, surgical treatment may be considered. Surgery generally consists of scapular stabilization and/or tendon transfers.

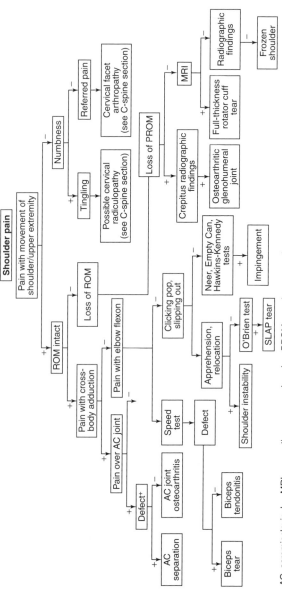

AC, acromioclavicular; MRI, magnetic resonance imaging; PROM, passive range of motion; ROM, range of motion; SLAP, superior labrum anterior and posterior.

Shoulder Pain

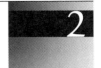

2

Red Flag Signs and Symptoms

Any of these signs and symptoms should prompt urgent evaluation and appropriate intervention:

Fevers
Chills
Hot, swollen joint
Progressive neurologic symptoms
Loss of pulses

IMPINGEMENT SYNDROME (ROTATOR CUFF TENDONITIS)

Background

The rotator cuff is made up of the SITS (*s*upraspinatus, *i*nfraspinatus, *t*eres minor, and *s*ubscapularis) muscles. Rotator cuff tendon impingement syndrome is perhaps the most common cause of shoulder pain seen by physicians. Impingement of the rotator cuff tendon occurs in the subacromial space. In this area, the rotator cuff tendon is impinged beneath the coracoacromial arch (which includes the coracoid process, coracoacromial ligament, acromion, and acromioclavicular joint capsule). In each case of impingement, muscle imbalances likely play a role. If the rotator cuff muscles and scapular stabilizers (e.g., trapezius, rhomboids, serratus anterior) muscles are properly conditioned, the cuff tendon will be better protected and less likely to be injured. When they are imbalanced or weak, the tendon is vulnerable, particularly with repetitive overhead activities.

Neer described this continuum of rotator cuff pathology with three stages. Stage I includes microtrauma that leads to edema and hemorrhage. Stage II leads to fibrosis of the tendon. In stage III, the tendon tears. Appreciating this continuum is useful to help us understand the importance of early and aggressive conservative care.

Subacromial bursitis is also often present with impingement syndrome. The subacromial bursa sits directly beneath the acromion where the tendon passes. Irritation of this bursa can lead to identical symptoms of impingement syndrome. In addition, because the causative factors are the same; because it can and often does lead to inflammation of the tendon; and because the treatment is virtually identical (the one exception is spelled out later in the treatment section), they are considered here as part of the same continuum of pathology.

Clinical Presentation

Patients typically present with complaints of gradual onset sharp superior, anterior, and/or lateral shoulder pain. The pain is exacerbated by overhead activities such as tennis, throwing sports, swimming, or weightlifting. Difficulty with everyday activities such as combing their hair, reaching for the back pocket, and putting on a shirt or bra is also characteristic of impingement syndrome.

If the shoulder pain has lasted for a few weeks or more, or if the pain has been recurring over a matter of years, the patient may note shoulder stiffness and/or weakness limiting daily activities such as carrying bags and picking up children. This is more indicative of shoulder impingement syndrome that has developed into a slight rotator cuff tear.

Physical Examination

Range of motion testing is usually unrestricted in patients, but a painful arc between 70 degrees to 120 degrees of shoulder abduction may be noted. A number of tests are specifically designed to test for impingement syndrome. Three good tests include the modified Hawkins-Kennedy test, Neer test, and Empty Can test. Each of these tests

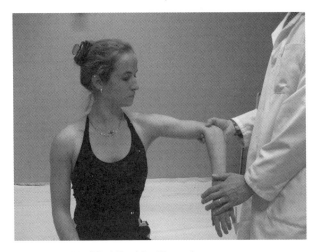

Figure 2.1 Modified Hawkins-Kennedy test.

seeks to reproduce the patient's symptoms by thrusting the rotator cuff complex into the undersurface of the coracoacromial arch.

In the modified Hawkins-Kennedy test (Fig. 2.1), the patient's arm is positioned with the elbow flexed to 90 degrees and the shoulder passively abducted to 90 degrees. The shoulder is then swiftly and firmly internally rotated. This procedure is repeated at various degrees of shoulder horizontal adduction ranging from 0 to 90 degrees of horizontal adduction.

In the Neer test (Fig. 2.2), the scapula is stabilized and the shoulder is internally rotated and passively flexed to 180 degrees. If symptoms are reproduced with the shoulder in internal rotation, it is considered a positive test. Pain in the shoulder occurs because the greater tuberosity of the humerus is brought in and abuts the tendon when the shoulder is in internal rotation and flexion causing irritation on an inflamed tendon.

In the Empty Can test (Fig. 2.3), the patient positions the shoulder in 90 degrees of abduction with 30 degrees of horizontal adduction. With the elbows extended and

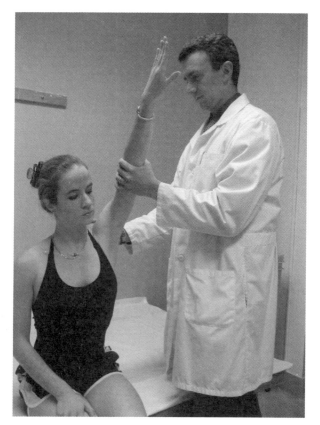

Figure 2.2 Neer test.

the patient's thumbs facing down (shoulder internal rotation), the patient then resists the examiner's downward force. The test is positive when pain is reproduced.

Diagnostic Studies

Radiographs should be obtained. Bigliani has described three different types of acromions. Type I is flat. Type II is curved. Type III is hooked. Impingement syndrome and

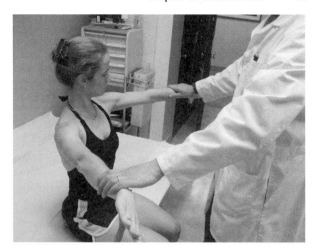

Figure 2.3   Empty Can test.

rotator cuff tear is much more likely if the acromion is a type II or III. Radiographs will also reveal the presence of a calcific deposit (see section on calcific tendonitis later) that may be causing impingement.

Magnetic resonance imaging (MRI) may be useful to evaluate a suspected rotator cuff tear. Ultrasound also may be useful for this purpose, but MRI remains the gold standard with a sensitivity of close to 100% for full tears.

The gold-standard diagnostic test for impingement syndrome is to perform impingement physical examination maneuvers and then inject lidocaine (or other anesthetic) into the subacromial space. After 5 minutes, the physical examination maneuvers are performed again and should be much less painful. Because the physical examination is typically diagnostic of impingement syndrome, the diagnostic injection is often used therapeutically as well and corticosteroid is also injected.

Treatment

The cornerstone of treatment for impingement syndrome is physical therapy that focuses on strengthening the rotator

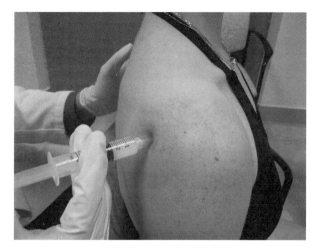

Figure 2.4 Subacromial steroid injection using posterior approach.

cuff muscles and scapular stabilizers. In addition, patients should be educated in proper posture and biomechanics. Ice, nonsteroidal anti-inflammatory drugs (NSAIDs), and activity modification are important treatment options.

If physical therapy and medications fail, or if symptoms severely limit activities of daily living on initial presentation, a subacromial corticosteroid injection is the treatment of choice. Although several potential approaches are possible, the authors favor a posterior approach (Fig. 2.4). After the area has undergone sterile preparation, a mixture of lidocaine and triamcinolone acetonide is injected into the subacromial space.

SUBACROMIAL STEROID INJECTION

A posterolateral approach is favored by the authors. After informed consent is obtained, identify the acromion. The authors favor using a 25-gauge, 1.5 inch needle, 40 mg of triamcinolone acetate, and 3 mL of 1% lidocaine. Mark a spot approximately 3 cm beneath the acromion. Sterilize this area using three iodine swabs and an alcohol pad. Using sterile technique, aim the needle parallel to the ground in the direction of the coracoid process (identified anteriorly by palpation). Always aspirate before injecting. If blood is found in the aspirate, reposition. There should be no aspirate in this injection. If resistance is felt, do not inject. Reposition and aspirate again. When there is no aspirate and the injectate flows smoothly, inject. Clean the iodine off with alcohol pads. Instruct the patient to dangle his or her arm toward the ground and move the shoulder through its range of motion (Codman exercises).

Recent studies have suggested that despite the apparent ease of this procedure, many practitioners do not reach the subacromial space. As a result, ultrasound guidance is suggested, and many practitioners are employing this technique. In addition, if ultrasound is used, the subacromial bursa can be visualized. If this bursa is inflamed, the physician can use the ultrasound to guide the needle directly into the bursa. Ultrasound guidance may one day become the standard of care. In the meantime, this is a simple injection procedure done in the office. It often alleviates the patient's pain.

Impingement syndrome is typically treated very successfully with nonsurgical care. If symptoms do persist for >6 to 12 months despite aggressive conservative care, however, surgical decompression of the subacromial space may be considered. This can be done arthroscopically or with open technique.

FULL-THICKNESS ROTATOR CUFF TEAR

Background

As mentioned in the previous section, Neer believed a rotator cuff tear is the culmination of a continuum of pathology seen in the shoulder. Although rotator cuff tears occur from chronic overuse, it can also tear from a sudden trauma. But the more common scenario is a weakened cuff tendon from years of microtrauma leading to inflammation and then fibrosis. Then, either the tendon just gradually tears or a small trauma puts the cuff "over the edge" and it simply fails.

Clinical Presentation

Usually a patient with a full-thickness rotator cuff tear presents with severe pain with major weakness and limited active range of motion. The pain in the shoulder may resolve over time, but range of motion never fully returns unless surgical repair is performed. Most of the difficulties patients complain of deal with any overhead movement.

Physical Examination

In a true rotator cuff tear, weakness is often present on examination. The drop arm test detects a full-thickness tear. In this test, the patient's arm is passively abducted to 90 degrees and then the patient is instructed to *slowly* lower the arm back to neutral. If a large tear is present, the patient's arm "drops" toward the ground. Testing the cuff muscles includes checking abduction (supraspinatus), internal rotation (subscapularis), and external rotation (infraspinatus and teres minor). Some physicians recommend testing the supraspinatus with the shoulder in internal rotation and during the first 30 degrees of abduction (with the scapula stabilized). This eliminates any abduction caused by deltoid contraction and helps isolate the rotator cuff complex.

Diagnostic Studies

The gold standard for assessing a full-thickness tear is an MRI. The MRI gives the surgeon information regarding the thickness of the tear and the presence of other injury that may have occurred during a traumatic event such as a biceps tear.

Radiograph may show narrowing of the subacromial space. One of the functions of the rotator cuff complex is to depress the humeral head to maintain glenohumeral articulation. If a tear occurs, the humeral head migrates superiorly, narrowing the subacromial space.

Arthrograms were commonly used in the past. In shoulder arthrography, dye is injected and a radiograph is taken to detect any leaks. If a leak is present this indicated a tear. With the advent of MRI, this imaging method is not as commonly used.

Ultrasound has recently become a reliable imaging tool for detecting rotator cuff tears. In the hands of a well-trained technician, the detection of a full-thickness tear with ultrasound can be as reliable as the other imaging methods.

Treatment

If a rotator cuff tear is present, treatment ranges from conservative to surgical repair. Partial thickness tears (<50% thickness) may be treated conservatively with physical therapy. If the partial tear is concomitant with impingement syndrome causing pain, a subacromial steroid injection may be helpful. If the tear does not respond to conservative treatment, arthroscopic debridement or subacromial decompression may be needed.

If the tear has >50% involvement, surgery may be indicated. The decision to undergo surgical repair depends on the patient's prior and expected function. If the patient is elderly, sedentary, and does not participate in much overhead activity, physical therapy to maximize function is the usual treatment choice. If the patient is a young carpenter who relies on overhead activities, surgical repair is the treatment of choice.

BICIPITAL TENDONITIS

Background

The biceps brachii has two heads. The short head arises from the tip of the coracoid process. The long head arises from the supraglenoid tubercle and superior labrum. The long head courses inferiorly between the greater and lesser humerus tubercles (in the bicipital groove) before joining the short head in the distal arm that inserts on the radial tuberosity of the radius. The biceps functions to flex the elbow, supinate the elbow, and depress the humeral head, and the short head flexes the shoulder. Many cases of bicipital tendonitis may be misdiagnosed as impingement syndrome because the two can present similarly. Of note, bicipital tendonitis and rotator cuff impingement syndrome can and sometimes do coexist.

Clinical Presentation

Pain is typically located in the anterior shoulder in the bicipital groove. Pain may refer to the entire shoulder or down the biceps tendon into the arm. Pain is aggravated with overhead activities and sometimes with carrying heavy loads with the elbow in flexion.

Physical Examination

The three important tests when evaluating for bicipital tendonitis are palpation, Speed test, and Yergason test.

Palpation of the biceps tendon is an important and sensitive way to assess for bicipital tendonitis. The tendon is often inflamed as it courses through the bicipital groove. The bicipital groove can be easily found by palpating the greater tuberosity of the shoulder and, with your other hand, passively internally and externally rotating the shoulder. The greater tuberosity will move out from under your finger. Medial to the greater tuberosity is the groove. Medial to the groove is the lesser tuberosity. Tenderness in the groove indicates potential tendonitis. Be sure to assess that this is the patient's "typical pain," however, and compare with the normal side because many people's bicipital tendon is tender in the groove. Also palpate the tendon more distally as it comes together with the short head of the biceps.

The Speed test (Fig. 2.5) is another good test for bicipital tendonitis. In this test, the patient flexes the shoulder to 90 degrees. The elbow is almost fully extended. Reproduction of the patient's symptoms with resisted shoulder flexion is indicative of bicipital tendonitis.

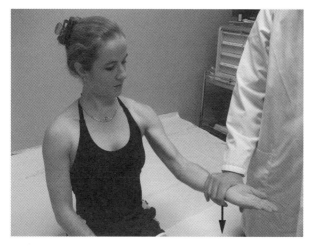

Figure 2.5   Speed test.

In the Yergason test (Fig. 2.6), the patient's elbow is flexed to 90 degrees and stabilized next to the thorax. The examiner then takes the patient's hand as if they are shaking hands. The examiner then tells the patient to turn their hand as if they were trying to show a bowl of soup, in essence asking the patient to supinate their forearm. Reproduction of pain symptoms with resisted supination indicates bicipital tendonitis.

Diagnostic Studies

Bicipital tendonitis is primarily a clinical diagnosis. Radiographs may be obtained to rule out a calcification or to assess bony structures.

Treatment

Ice, NSAIDs, activity modification, and physical therapy are effective in treating this condition. A steroid and anesthetic injection into the tendon sheath (*never the tendon*) is also very effective (Fig. 2.7). Ultrasound guidance for this injection may be helpful.

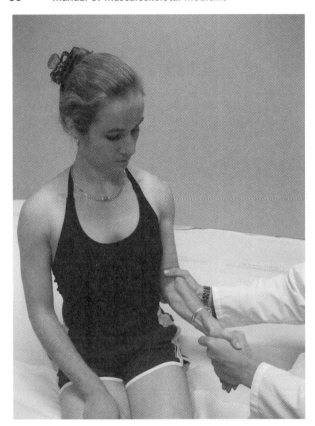

Figure 2.6   Yergason test.

BICIPITAL TENDONITIS INJECTION

After informed consent is obtained, identify the point of maximal tenderness along the biceps tendon. This point is often in the bicipital groove, located between the greater and lesser humeral tuberosities. This can be identified easily by having the patient internally and externally rotate the shoulder as the examiner palpates

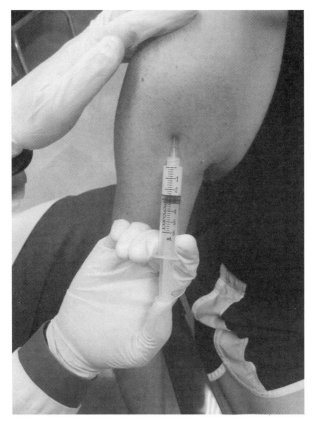

Figure 2.7 Bicipital tendon injection.

the tuberosity moving underneath his or her thumb. The authors favor using a 25-gauge, 1.5 inch needle, 40 mg of triamcinolone acetate, and 3 mL of 1% lidocaine. Mark a spot approximately 3 cm inferior to the point of maximal tenderness along the tendon. Sterilize this area using three iodine swabs and an alcohol pad. Using sterile technique, the needle is aimed at approximately a 45-degree angle to the tendon. Always aspirate before injecting. If blood is found in the aspirate, reposition. There should be no aspirate in this injection. If resistance is felt, do not inject. Resistance indicates that you may be in the tendon. *Never inject into the tendon.* Instead, back off the tendon, reposition, and aspirate again. When there is no aspirate and the injectate flows *smoothly*, with no resistance, inject. Clean the iodine off with alcohol pads.

BICEPS TENDON RUPTURE

Background

When the biceps tendon ruptures, it usually occurs proximally at the tendon-glenoid labrum junction affecting the long head of the biceps.

Clinical Presentation

Patients may complain of a sudden, sharp pain in the anterior shoulder and audible snap at the time of rupture. Typically, they have been lifting a relatively heavy weight. Patients may note a quick development of ecchymosis and visible bulging of their lower arm. Patients often are between 40 and 60 years of age and report a history of recurring shoulder pain in the past. Other patients may report only mild soreness in their shoulder, or be asymptomatic except they notice a visible and palpable mass in their shoulder or arm. They also may notice bruising in their arm.

Physical Examination

Ecchymosis is often apparent over the anterior shoulder and arm. A bulge may be evident in the lower arm (resulting from retraction of the biceps after rupture) and can be accentuated by having the patient flex the elbow. The bicipital groove may appear hollow or "scooped out" with the absence of the tendon. Pain and weakness may be noted with resisted elbow flexion. If only a partial tear is present, the Yergason test and Speed test will help identify them as they reveal bicipital pain and instability.

Diagnostic Studies

Biceps tendon rupture is primarily a clinical diagnosis. Radiographs may be obtained to rule out fracture or evaluate bony spurs, but they are not generally needed. Ultrasound may be useful for evaluation. MRI is the gold standard for diagnosis and should be obtained if surgery is being contemplated.

Treatment

Treatment for this disorder depends on the patient's needs and expectations. Patients treated with aggressive conservative therapy, including physical therapy and ice, typically regain full range of motion and most elbow flexion strength. Supination power may be somewhat decreased (about 20% from baseline). Activities of daily living and most recreational activities should not be greatly impacted. In younger, athletic patients, patients who perform hard manual labor and require full strength, or in patients with persistent shoulder pain, surgical repair may be indicated. Prior to surgery, an MRI should be obtained to evaluate extent of injury and also evaluate for possible concomitant tear of the rotator cuff tendon or other shoulder pathology. Another indication for surgery is cosmetic deformity from the biceps rupture.

SUPERIOR LABRAL ANTERIOR POSTERIOR LESION

Background

The glenoid labrum is made of a cartilaginous lining of the glenoid fossa. Its purpose is to deepen the glenoid and provide stability for the shoulder. The biceps tendon attaches to the superior aspect of this labrum. Injuries to the labrum are often caused by chronic repetitive stress, resulting in fraying of the labrum, or frank tears from sudden trauma. When the tear in the labrum involves the superior aspect of the labrum, it is termed a SLAP (superior labrum anterior and posterior) lesion. Many physicians believe a SLAP lesion is a result of traction from the long head of the biceps tendon pulling on the labrum.

Clinical Presentation

Patients typically present with shoulder pain that is worsened with overhead activities. The pain may be anterior or may present as a "deep ache" within the shoulder. Sometimes the patient may report "popping" or "catching." However, in general, the history for a patient with a SLAP lesion may sound very similar to impingement syndrome. Occasionally, a patient may report falling onto an outstretched arm, precipitating the symptoms.

Physical Examination

One of the most important physical examination findings in a patient with a SLAP lesion is the *absence* of impingement signs. Of course, a SLAP lesion can coexist with impingement syndrome. But a patient with an isolated SLAP lesion should have negative impingement tests (modified Hawkins-Kennedy, Neer, Empty Can). The O'Brien test (Fig. 2.8) does not have strong sensitivity or specificity. Nevertheless, many physicians find it the most useful for physical examination diagnosis. In this test, the patient flexes the shoulder to 90 degrees with the elbow in full extension. The arm is then adducted 15 degrees across the body. The shoulder is internally rotated so the thumb points down at the ground. The physician then applies an inferiorly directed force on the patient's arm while the patient resists. This procedure is repeated with the patient's arm in external rotation and the thumb pointed toward the ceiling. The test is positive if the patient experiences

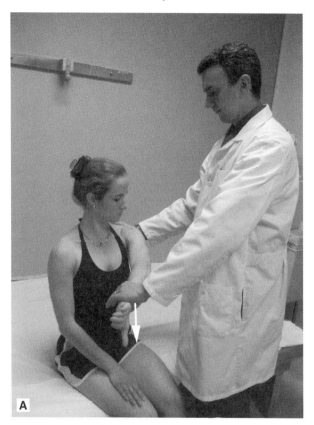

Figure 2.8 **(A)** O'Brien test.

pain with resistance when the shoulder is internally rotated and is pain free when the shoulder is in external rotation. In addition, the pain must be typical of the patient's pain and experienced *within* the shoulder.

Diagnostic Studies

Radiographs should be obtained but will not reveal the SLAP lesion. They will, however, reveal any bony abnormalities. MRI without contrast has <50% sensitivity. The test of

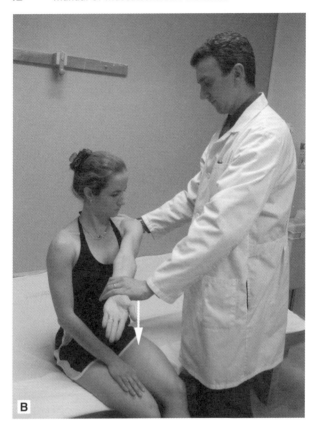

Figure 2.8 **(B)** O' Brien test *(continued)*.

choice is MR arthrography. This is a more invasive test that involves the injection of contrast into the shoulder prior to MRI. The sensitivity and specificity is only approximately 90%, but it is the best imaging test currently available.

Treatment

Physical therapy that focuses on scapular stabilization and rotator cuff strengthening is first-line treatment.

Posterior capsule stretching is also helpful. Activity modification including limiting overhead activities that produce pain is also recommended. NSAIDs can also be used. An intra-articular steroid injection under fluoroscopic or ultrasound guidance can also be helpful to quiet the inflammation and facilitate participation with therapy. Resistant cases may require arthroscopic surgical intervention to debride and possibly repair the lesion. A patient with concomitant biceps tear or biceps tendonitis may benefit from a biceps tenodesis in which the biceps tendon is detached from where it inserts in the labrum and reattached to a different site. This reduces the constant pulling on that part of the labrum and may provide more lasting relief.

SHOULDER INSTABILITY/SHOULDER DISLOCATION

Background

The glenoid fossa is relatively shallow and the capsule relatively loose when compared with other joints such as the hip. Because of this, the shoulder has a broad range of motion, but in return for this flexibility, it is also prone to instability. In fact, the shoulder is the most commonly dislocated joint in the body. Instability refers to recurring painful subluxation that is a partial dislocation of the humeral head from the glenoid. Instability can result from macrotrauma, repetitive microtrauma, deconditioned rotator cuff muscles, a torn long head of the biceps tendon (responsible in part for humeral head depression), or a combination thereof. The most common form of instability is multidirectional and usually atraumatic.

Dislocation is seen when no contact between the articular surface of the humeral head and the glenoid fossa occurs. Dislocations usually occur from a traumatic event forcing the shoulder to disarticulate in one direction. The most common form of dislocation is anterior inferior. Posterior dislocation can also occur but is much less common.

Clinical Presentation

Patients with anterior instability typically present with complaints of shoulder pain and the feeling that the shoulder is "slipping out" or "unstable." If the instability began with a trauma, the patient may recall a significant fall, being tackled, or other trauma. Younger patients may report a fall onto an outstretched hand. In some patients, the symptoms may have come on more gradually. Patients with anterior instability relate that their symptoms are worst with their shoulder in abduction and external rotation such as reaching behind their head or when throwing a ball.

Patients with multidirectional instability report more vague symptoms. They have a feeling of instability, pain, or feeling hesitant when performing activities with their shoulder. Multidirectional instability is rarely the result of a single trauma.

Patients with posterior instability usually report symptoms that began immediately after a major trauma such as being hit by a car or having a seizure.

Physical Examination

If the dislocation is acute, the patient will have recently suffered a trauma and be holding the shoulder in the neutral position and the examination will be limited because any movement of the shoulder will be very painful. If the arm has been acutely dislocated posteriorly (which, as mentioned, is rare), the arm will be held in adduction and internal rotation. As always, a thorough neurovascular examination should be performed. The axillary vessels and the axillary nerve can sometimes be injured with a dislocation and may result in temporary shoulder abduction weakness and paresthesias over the deltoid.

If the shoulder complaints lack any history of trauma, a few tests can be used to determine the presence of instability. The anterior apprehension test (Fig. 2.9A) is good for detecting anterior instability. In this test, the patient lies supine on the examining table with the involved shoulder hanging off the table. The examiner takes the shoulder and passively abducts the shoulder to 90 degrees and then

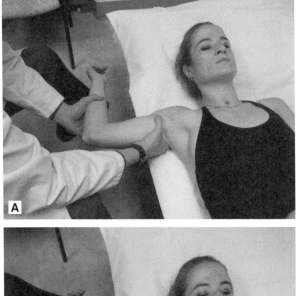

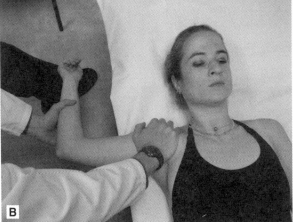

Figure 2.9 (A) Anterior apprehension test. (B) Relocation test.

slowly externally rotates the arm using the wrist and elbow as a fulcrum. If the patient reports any apprehension while the arm is externally rotated, such as a feeling that the shoulder is going to "pop" or "slip" out, the test is positive. Pain may also be elicited, but this is less specific. If the apprehension sign is positive, then perform the relocation test. In this test, you perform the same maneuver, except this time you simultaneously apply a posteriorly directed pressure with the palm of your hand on the anterior shoulder (Fig. 2.9B). This should keep the humeral head within the glenoid fossa and reduce the patient's apprehension.

The sulcus sign is another good test and assesses for inferior shoulder laxity. In this test, the patient is seated with the arm relaxed and hanging at the side. The examiner applies inferior traction to the patient's shoulder. If this maneuver creates an inferior subluxation or increased space between the humeral head and acromion when compared with the asymptomatic side, it is considered positive.

A good test for posterior instability is to have the patient lie supine, hold the arm flexed to 90 degrees, and place an inferiorly directed force (Fig. 2.10). Compare with the asymptomatic side. If there is greater laxity on one side than the other, the test is considered positive.

When assessing for laxity, make note of the patient's overall laxity. A good quick assessment for this is to ask the patient to touch his thumb backward against the volar aspect of his forearm. Extend the elbow, wrist, metacarpal-phalangeal,

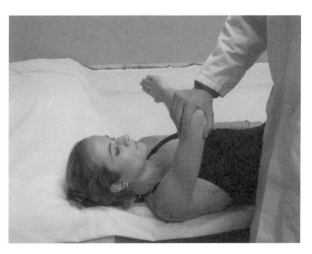

Figure 2.10   Posterior instability test.

and distal interphalangeal joints. Generalized joint laxity is important to note because it will affect the degree of laxity you can expect on the shoulder examination and also because patients with increased overall ligamentous laxity are more likely to have multidirectional instability.

Diagnostic Studies

Radiographs should be obtained. A Hill-Sachs lesion, a compression fracture of the posterior humeral head indicative of an anterior dislocation, may be seen. It occurs as the soft base of the posterior head is compressed into the relatively hard anterior glenoid (Fig. 2.11).

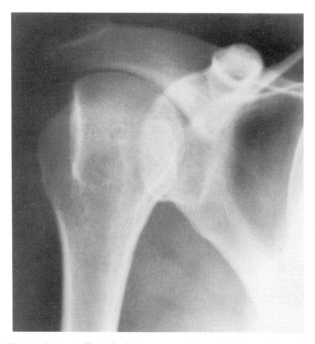

Figure 2.11 Hill-Sachs lesion on radiograph. (From Chew F, Roberts, C. *Musculoskeletal Imaging: A Teaching File*. 2nd ed. Philadelphia, Pa: Lippincott Williams & Wilkins, 2006, with permission.)

MRI is useful in detecting a Bankart lesion, which is a tear of the anteroinferior glenoid labrum. When this is present, surgical stabilization may be necessary.

Treatment

In general, the sooner an acute anterior dislocation is reduced, the better. There are many protocols for reducing an acute dislocation. Radiographs may be required prior to reduction depending on the presentation, patient, and comfort level of the physician. In the Stimson technique, the patient lies prone on the table with the dislocated arm hanging over the side. The physician's assistant provides downward traction on the arm (alternatively a 5- to 15-pound weight can be tied to the patient's arm). The physician then places his or her left thumb on the patient's acromion and fingers wrap around the front of the humeral head. As the muscles relax and the arm is pulled downward, the physician gently maneuvers the humeral head caudally, reducing it.

Following reduction of an acute dislocation, the patient should be enrolled in a structured physical therapy program that focuses on rotator cuff strengthening and periscapular stabilization to help prevent future recurrence.

In patients with a *t*raumatic *u*nidirectional instability with a *B*ankart lesion (tear of the anteroinferior glenoid labrum), *s*urgery is often indicated (**TUBS**).

*A*traumatic instability that is *m*ultidirectional and *b*ilateral responds very well to *r*ehabilitation therapy. When surgery is required, an *i*nferior capsular shift is the surgical procedure of choice (AMBRI). The rehabilitation therapy here should focus on rotator cuff strengthening and periscapular stabilization.

GLENOHUMERAL ARTHRITIS

Background

Glenohumeral arthritis is not nearly as common as hip and knee arthritis. Nevertheless, it is a cause of shoulder pain that should be included in the differential diagnosis.

Increased age is a significant risk factor (patients are typically >50 years). History of injury to the joint and muscle imbalances surrounding the joint may also contribute to the development of shoulder arthritis. By far the predominant form of shoulder arthritis is osteoarthritis. Osteoarthritis typically presents unilaterally, whereas rheumatoid arthritis typically presents with bilateral, symmetric complaints and systemic symptoms.

Clinical Presentation

Patients typically complain of vague and diffuse shoulder pain. The symptoms have often gradually progressed. Initially, pain is present only with shoulder exertion. As the disease progresses, pain occurs with minimal shoulder movement. Later in the disease, pain may be present at rest and at nighttime. Patients may also note decreased range of motion (primarily from pain and disuse).

Physical Examination

Atrophy of the cuff muscles and deltoid may be noted on inspection and palpation. The shoulder may be tender to deep palpation. Range of motion may be restricted. With the patient supine, passive grinding of the humerus into the glenoid may reproduce painful symptoms. Crepitus may be noted with shoulder internal and external rotation and/or flexion.

Diagnostic Studies

Radiographs should be obtained and characteristically reveal joint space narrowing, osteophytes, erosion of the glenoid, subchondral cyst formation, and other signs of osteoarthritis (Fig. 2.12). Severity of osteoarthritis seen on radiographs does not necessarily correlate with symptoms.

If rheumatoid arthritis is the cause of symptoms, erosions and osteopenia may be present.

Computed tomography and MRI are not generally indicated unless obtained to rule out other pathology.

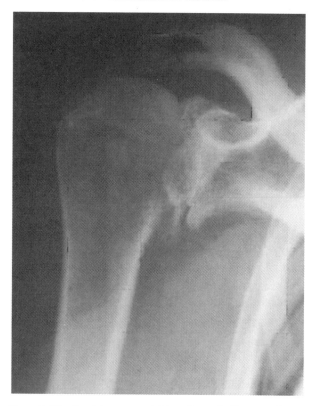

Figure 2.12   Shoulder osteoarthritis radiograph. (From Moskowitz et al. *Osteoarthritis: Diagnosis and Medical/Surgical Management.* 4th ed. Philadelphia, Pa: Lippincott Williams & Wilkins, 2007, with permission.)

Treatment

Because severity of symptoms does not necessarily corre-late with severity of radiographic findings, remember to always treat the patient, not the film. As with osteoarthri-tis in other parts of the body, the sooner that conservative care is implemented, the better the outcome. Patients should begin a program of structured physical therapy that focuses on rotator cuff strengthening, scapular stabilization, and stretching. Once the patient has learned the exercises, they should be continued as part of a home exercise program.

Oral supplementation with glucosamine and chondroitin sulfate may be helpful. NSAIDs and other pain killers may be necessary to permit the patient to participate in therapy. Their use for long-term treatment is not advisable because of the side effects.

Intra-articular injections of corticosteroid can be very effective in treating osteoarthritis. Intra-articular injections of hyaluronic acid (such as is done in the knee) are currently undergoing investigation for use in the shoulder. It is not currently the standard of care, but its use does appear promising for this purpose. All intra-articular shoulder injections should ideally be done under fluoroscopic or ultrasound guidance.

A suprascapular nerve block may also be effective in reducing pain and allowing the patient to participate in therapy more adequately (Fig. 2.13).

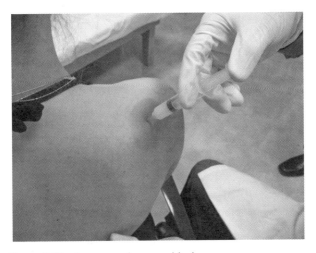

Figure 2.13   Suprascapular nerve block.

SUPRASCAPULAR NERVE BLOCK

The suprascapular nerve runs through the suprascapular notch. After informed consent is obtained, identify the midpoint of the spine of the scapula. The authors favor using a 25-gauge, 1.5 inch needle, 40 mg of triamcinolone acetate, and 3 mL of 1% lidocaine. Mark a spot approximately 2 to 3 cm superior to the midpoint of the spine of the scapula. Sterilize this area using three iodine swabs and an alcohol pad. Using sterile technique, aim the needle parallel to the ground anteriorly until bony contact is made. Back off slightly, aspirate, and inject. If blood is found in the aspirate, reposition before injecting. There should be no aspirate in this injection. Clean the iodine off with alcohol pads.

For patients with advanced shoulder osteoarthritis that interferes with quality of life and who are resistant to conservative care, surgery may be an option. When needed, the most common and generally preferred form of surgery for shoulder osteoarthritis is total joint replacement. In younger patients interested in continuing to lift heavy loads and stay very active, a hemiarthroplasty may be more appropriate. In patients with damaged muscles or tendons that are incapable of supporting a replacement, a shoulder arthrodesis may be appropriate.

ACROMIOCLAVICULAR JOINT ARTHRITIS

Background

The acromioclavicular (AC) joint is a common area to become arthritic. A history of shoulder instability and/or AC joint separation or trauma makes it more likely that the patient will one day develop AC arthritis.

Clinical Presentation

Patients typically present with complaints of gradually developing anterior shoulder pain and/or pain over the AC joint. Pain is exacerbated by shoulder movements, particularly movements that involve shoulder adduction.

Physical Examination

The patient may have pain to palpation over the AC joint. A typical and important finding is the cross-arm test, also known as the scarf test. In this test, the examiner passively adducts the patient's arm across the chest. When pain is reproduced, the test is positive. The AC squeeze test (Fig. 2.14) is another test that indicates the presence of AC joint pathology. This is performed with the examiner placing the base of the palm of one hand over the spine of the scapula and the other over the clavicle. The examiner then interlocks fingers and squeezes. Pain over the AC joint indicates AC joint pathology. Another important finding to note is the O'Brien test (see section on SLAP lesion and Fig. 2.9 for details of this test). If this test reproduces pain over the AC joint and *not* in the shoulder, the pathology is likely coming from the AC joint itself.

Diagnostic Studies

Radiographs should be obtained and may reveal joint space narrowing and possibly other findings of osteoarthritis.

Treatment

Conservative care consists of NSAIDs, ice, and physical therapy. Topical analgesics may also be helpful because of the superficiality of the joint. A corticosteroid injection may be performed and often provides significant relief. The use of an AC joint brace may also be useful to stabilize and provide relief. The brace is especially useful in athletes or laborers who continue to have high shoulder demands.

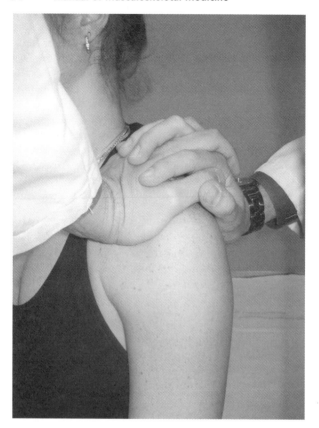

Figure 2.14   Acromioclavicular squeeze test.

If symptoms interfere with quality of life and persist despite aggressive conservative therapy, surgical options include removing the distal portion of the clavicle. The space fills in with scar tissue and the patient should have full use of the AC joint after recovery and physical therapy.

ADHESIVE CAPSULITIS (FROZEN SHOULDER)

Background

The pathophysiologic basis for frozen shoulder remains debated and under investigation. It typically affects women from 40 to 70 years of age. Diabetes (type I in particular) is a major risk factor. Other risk factors include hypothyroidism, Parkinson disease, cardiac disease, tumors, and shoulder injury. Overall the most common cause is idiopathic.

Clinical Presentation

Patients typically report a history of insidious, dull, achy shoulder pain that begins at night. The pain then becomes apparent with small shoulder movements such as putting on a shirt, brushing hair, and reaching for a wallet in the back pocket. The pain progresses to pain even at rest. As the pain intensifies and becomes more constant, the patient begins to note a loss of range of motion. This is sometimes known as the "freezing stage" and may last from 1 to 9 months post onset of symptoms.

During the "frozen stage," patients note a gradual improvement in pain, but the stiffness and loss of range of motion remains. This stage may last from 5 to 18 months after the onset of symptoms.

During the "thawing stage," patients note an improvement of stiffness and generally regain most of their lost range of motion. Patients tend to plateau in their recovery approximately 2 to 3 years after the onset of symptoms if no treatment is instituted or treatment is not effective.

Physical Examination

On examination, in the early "freezing stage," the most pronounced finding may be pain with end range of motion. Diffuse tenderness over the shoulder may also be present. Typically, patients lose range of motion in external rotation and abduction first. Flexion is often relatively preserved.

Diagnostic Studies

Radiographs are routine to rule out other pathology. MR arthrogram is not routine but may be obtained to confirm the diagnosis.

Treatment

Physical therapy that focuses on gentle stretching exercises is indicated. Also indicated are NSAIDs, other analgesics, and moist heat, particularly prior to stretching. Ice may be used after stretching.

An intra-articular injection of corticosteroid, particularly if done in the freezing stage, may be helpful. This should be done under ultrasound or fluoroscopic guidance.

A suprascapular nerve block (see Fig. 2.13 along with box) is helpful for certain patients with frozen shoulder. Given the very low risks of the procedure when done correctly, this is also a good alternative.

Some physicians advocate glenohumeral manipulation under general anesthesia during the frozen stage. However, studies have indicated that patients with frozen shoulder may do better if *not* manipulated in this manner. Given the overall highly favorable outcome of the natural history of frozen shoulder, this practice is discouraged. Similarly, surgical options have significant adverse potential reactions and do not improve outcome significantly.

ACROMIOCLAVICULAR SEPARATION

Background

Acromioclavicular (AC) injuries commonly refer from a trauma such as a fall onto the shoulder. They are classified into six types based on severity of injury and degree of separation (Fig. 2.15). In type I, the AC joint ligaments undergo a minor sprain but the coracoclavicular (CC) ligaments are intact. In type II, the AC ligaments are torn, the joint capsule is ruptured, and the CC ligaments undergo

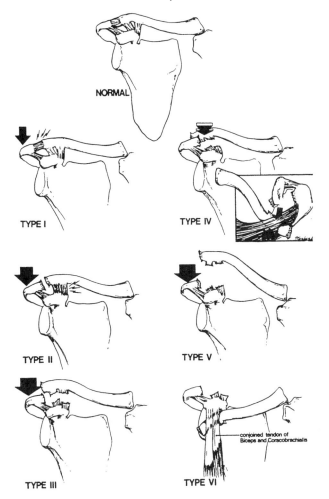

Figure 2.15 Acromioclavicular separation. (From Safran MR, MeKeag, DB, VanCamp SP. *Manual of Sports Medicine*. Philadelphia, Pa: Lippincott-Raven, 1998, with permission.)

a minor sprain, resulting in minimal separation of the clavicle from the acromion. In type III, the AC and CC ligaments are completely torn and the joint capsule is ruptured, resulting in complete separation of the clavicle from the acromion. Types IV through VI are rare. Types IV and V involve detachment of the deltoid and trapezius. Briefly, type IV also involves posterior displacement of the clavicle. Types V and VI involve the clavicle being displaced superiorly and behind the biceps tendon, respectively.

Clinical Presentation

Patients report a recent history of trauma, such as a collision in football, martial arts strike, fall onto an adducted shoulder, or motor vehicle accident that immediately precipitated the symptoms. Patients typically experience diffuse shoulder pain that is exacerbated with lifting or moving the shoulder. In patients with AC separation type III and higher, patients notice a deformity of their AC joint.

Physical Examination

Patients tend to present with their arm in an adducted position. Ecchymosis and abrasions may be present over the area secondary to the trauma. Palpation of the AC joint reveals tenderness and, depending on the type of injury, displacement of the clavicle (≥type II). Swelling may also be evident. Abduction, passive and active, is likely to be painful. The cross-arm test in which the patient's affected arm is passively adducted across his chest is also likely to reproduce pain.

It is important to perform a thorough neurovascular examination to rule out brachial plexus injury, which, though rare, may occur with this injury.

Diagnostic Studies

Radiographs of both shoulders should be obtained. Weighted radiographs using a 10- to 15-pound weight strapped to each wrist can also be used to aid in the visualization.

In type I injuries, radiographs are normal.

In type II injuries, radiographs reveal subluxation of the AC joint of <1 cm and normal CC space.

In type III injuries, radiographs reveal >1 cm of AC joint space subluxation and complete displacement of the clavicle with <25% to 100% widening of the CC space.

In type IV through VI injuries, the AC joint has >1 cm of subluxation, widening of the CC, and the clavicle is displaced posteriorly through the trapezius (type IV), superiorly into a subcutaneous position (type V), or inferiorly beneath the coracoid (type VI).

Ultrasound and/or MRI may be helpful in delineating concomitant soft tissue injury. In competitive athletes, MRI should be obtained, particularly if surgery is being contemplated.

Treatment

Types I and II AC joint separations can be treated nonsurgically with ice, analgesics, and a sling for a few days. After type I injuries, assuming resolution of symptoms and return to pain-free full range of motion, athletes can usually return to their sport within 2 weeks. After type II injuries, assuming asymptomatic with full range of motion, athletes must stay in the sling for up to 2 weeks and can generally return to their sport within 2 months.

Treatment for type III separation remains somewhat controversial. Some physicians believe nonoperative care offers the best outcomes, whereas others favor a more aggressive surgical approach, particularly in a patient who does a lot of manual heavy labor.

Types IV through VI require surgical evaluation and, typically, open reduction and internal fixation (ORIF).

After treatment for all types, patients should undergo a stretching and strengthening physical therapy program. In addition, athletes returning to contact sports, such as football or ice hockey, may benefit from an AC joint brace or special padding available to help cushion the AC joint in future collisions.

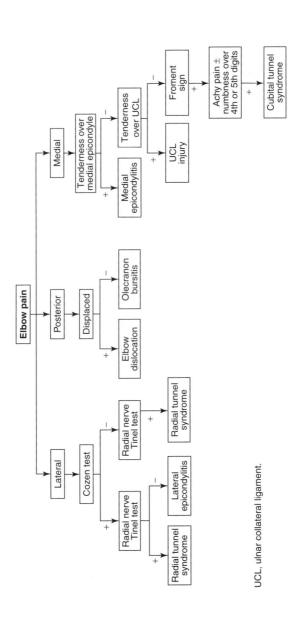

UCL, ulnar collateral ligament.

Elbow Pain

3

Red Flag Signs and Symptoms

Any of these signs and symptoms should prompt urgent evaluation and appropriate intervention:

Fevers
Chills
Hot, swollen joint
Progressive neurologic symptoms
Loss of pulses

LATERAL EPICONDYLITIS (TENNIS ELBOW)

Background

Despite the fact that many people who do not play tennis get this disorder, the term *tennis elbow* is still popularly used. Lateral epicondylitis itself turns out to be a misnomer because histologic studies reveal that tendinosis (fibrosis), not *itis* (inflammation) may be the underlying mechanism of the pathology. Nevertheless, the term *lateral epicondylitis* has persisted.

Overuse injuries with poor mechanics or ill-fitting equipment (inappropriate racket grip size, overly tight racket string tension, repetitive turning of a screwdriver) are contributing factors, as is a lack of muscle conditioning prior to these activities.

Clinical Presentation

Patients typically are 40 to 50 years of age and present with lateral elbow pain that occurs when performing activities such as lifting, shaking hands, or any other activity that requires repetitive forearm pronation and supination. As the pathology progresses, patients may relate pain with minimal activities such as opening a door and holding utensils. Because of this pain-limiting function, patients sometimes complain of "weakness."

Physical Examination

Localized tenderness is identified slightly distal to the lateral epicondyle at the common extensor origin. Resisted wrist extension typically elicits pain (Mill test) (Fig. 3.1). Passive wrist flexion with the elbow in extension may also elicit the patient's pain. Resisted extension of the third digit with the elbow in extension may also reproduce symptoms (although this can also be positive in radial tunnel syndrome). Resisted supination of the forearm is also typically painful. One way to test this is by shaking hands with the patient and applying a pronating force (making the patient supinate to resist).

Another good test is to stabilize the patient's elbow and palpate the lateral epicondyle as the patient pronates and

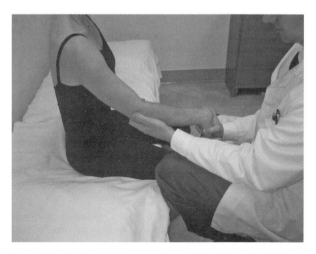

Figure 3.1   Resisted wrist extension typically elicits pain (Mill test).

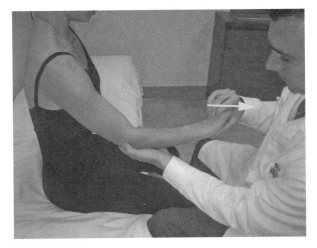

Figure 3.2 The Cozen test is another good test for lateral epicondylitis. Stabilize the patient's elbow and palpate the lateral epicondyle as the patient pronates and extends the wrist against resistance.

extends the wrist against resistance (Cozen test) (Fig. 3.2). Reproduction of symptoms is characteristic of lateral epicondylitis. This test can be done with the elbow flexed or extended. It may be more sensitive when the elbow is extended.

Diagnostic Studies

Radiographs are not always obtained but may be ordered to rule out other pathologies such as a loose body, fracture, or arthritis.

Treatment

Initial treatment consists of decreasing the pain and inflammation (inflammation may not be the underlying cause, but it does appear to be a factor) and removing or modifying the offending activity.

Ice is a terrific anti-inflammatory agent in this superficial condition. Anti-inflammatory creams can also be beneficial. Nonsteroidal anti-inflammatory drugs (NSAIDs) may be helpful.

An injection of anesthetic and corticosteroid (with care *not* to inject into the tendon) can be very helpful to speed recovery (Fig. 3.3). Sometimes the injection needs to be repeated (but should not be performed more than three times).

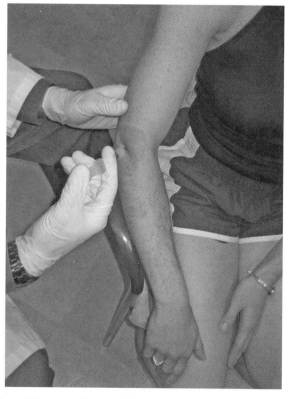

Figure 3.3   Lateral epicondylitis injection.

LATERAL EPICONDYLITIS INJECTION

After informed consent is obtained, identify the lateral epicondyle. The authors favor using a 25-gauge, 1.5 inch needle, 20 mg of triamcinolone acetate, and 1 mL of 1% lidocaine. Mark the point of maximal tenderness over the lateral epicondyle. Sterilize this area using three iodine swabs and an alcohol pad. Using sterile technique, aim the needle perpendicular into the point of maximal tenderness. Always aspirate before injecting. If blood is found in the aspirate, reposition. There should be no aspirate in this injection. If resistance is felt, do not inject. Resistance could indicate that the needle is in the tendon. *Never inject directly into the tendon.* Reposition and aspirate again. When there is no aspirate and the injectate flows smoothly, inject. Clean the iodine off with alcohol pads. Note that some physicians favor using 40 mg of triamcinolone acetate. In the authors' experience, 20 mg is sufficient.

Modifying equipment may be all that is necessary to remove the offending agent. Changing racket size or string tension and using an electric screwdriver are two examples. An epicondylar strap worn beneath the elbow may be helpful when lifting heavy loads is unavoidable.

Physical therapy that focuses on gentle stretching and strengthening should also be used. In the acute phase, modalities such as ultrasound and soft tissue mobilization can be employed.

Most patients (>95%) heal completely with aggressive conservative care. In the rare refractory case, surgical debridement of the tendinosis with decortication of the lateral epicondyle is an option.

RADIAL TUNNEL SYNDROME

Background

Radial tunnel syndrome is sometimes called "resistant tennis elbow" because the symptoms may be so similar to tennis elbow that the two are often confused. The diagnosis should be considered based on history and physical examination and also in patients diagnosed with lateral epicondylitis who have failed to respond to aggressive conservative therapy. Some physicians believe the two conditions may coexist in up to 5% of patients. In this syndrome, the radial nerve is compressed at the arcade of Frohse (which is at the elbow in the superior portion of the supinator) or in the inferior portion of the supinator muscle. Trauma can cause the syndrome, as can repetitive, forceful pronation and supination. At the site of compression, the radial nerve has branched into the posterior interosseus nerve, which is a purely motor nerve.

Clinical Presentation

Patients typically present with pain over the lateral epicondyle. As with lateral epicondylitis, the patient's pain is worsened with wrist extension and repetitive gripping and squeezing. Helpful distinguishing features of radial tunnel syndrome as opposed to lateral epicondylitis include night pain and pain that sometimes radiates over the forearm. In addition, the locus of pain is slightly distal to that of lateral epicondylitis. Occasionally, the pain refers to the dorsum of the hand. There are no sensory deficits (e.g., numbness) because only the posterior interosseous nerve is affected, which is a purely motor nerve. Patients do not complain of weakness in most cases. Weakness, if present, would include first digit and metacarpophalangeal (MCP) extension. Patients are able to extend their wrist but may have radial deviation.

Physical Examination

The middle finger test in which the middle finger is extended against resistance is likely to be positive in radial tunnel syndrome *and* in patients with lateral epicondylitis. One way to distinguish radial tunnel syndrome from lateral epicondylitis is to perform a Tinel test by tapping approximately 3 inches distal to the lateral epicondyle over the course of the radial nerve. Reproduction of pain signifies possible radial tunnel syndrome. Strength testing is generally normal. If weakness is present, severe compression should be suspected and weakness may be detected with extension of the first digit and MCPs (interphalangeal joint extension is intact). Radial deviation on extension may be present.

Diagnostic Studies

Electromyelography/nerve conduction velocity (EMG/NCV) studies may be performed to evaluate for radial tunnel syndrome, but this test has a high false-negative rate for this condition.

Treatment

Treatment consists of ice, relative rest (avoiding the offending activity if possible), and physical therapy. Wearing a lightweight plastic splint at night to reduce mobility of the elbow may help reduce unwanted supination and pronation while the muscles are relaxed during sleep. This may give the nerve an opportunity to heal. An injection of anesthetic and cortisone over the site of entrapment may be diagnostic and therapeutic. In severe cases, or recalcitrant cases, operative decompression may be necessary.

MEDIAL EPICONDYLITIS (GOLFER'S ELBOW)

Background

As with lateral epicondylitis, medial epicondylitis is a misnomer. The pathologic process is more tendinosis than tendonitis. Nevertheless, there is an inflammatory component. Medial epicondylitis is also called "golfer's elbow," but of course people other than golfers also are afflicted. The site of tendinosis is on the common tendinous origin of the flexor and pronator muscles slightly anterior and distal to the medial epicondyle.

Clinical Presentation

Patients are often 40 to 50 years of age and complain of medial epicondyle pain. The pain is exacerbated with activities that involve active forearm pronation and wrist flexion such as occurs when swinging a golf club, applying topspin in a tennis shot, using a screwdriver, and bowling. As the disease progresses, pain becomes more pronounced with less vigorous activities such as shaking hands.

If there is numbness or tingling extending into the medial forearm and fourth or fifth digits, ulnar nerve involvement should be suspected and interrogated for possible cubital tunnel syndrome.

Physical Examination

Tenderness is elicited just distal and anterior to the medial epicondyle. With the forearm pronated, wrist flexion against resistance typically reproduces painful symptoms (Fig. 3.4).

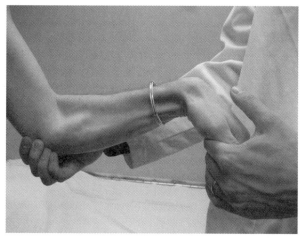

Figure 3.4   Medial epicondylitis test.

Diagnostic Studies

Radiographs are not always necessary but may be obtained to rule out arthritis, osteochondral lesions, and other bony lesions.

Treatment

Initial treatment consists of decreasing the pain and inflammation and removing or modifying the offending activity.

Ice may be used as a potent anti-inflammatory agent in this superficial condition. Anti-inflammatory creams can also be beneficial. NSAIDs may be helpful.

An injection of anesthetic and corticosteroid (with care *not* to inject into the tendon) can be very helpful to speed recovery (Fig. 3.5). Sometimes the injection needs to be repeated (but should not be performed more than three times).

Modifying activities and equipment (e.g., an electric screwdriver) is needed to relieve the constant stresses on the flexor/pronator muscles and tendon. A lateral epicondylitis strap can actually be placed anteromedially on the forearm over the flexor pronator mass.

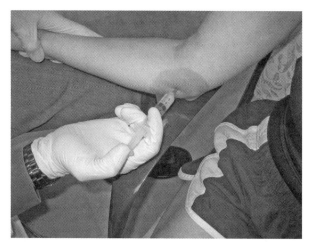

Figure 3.5   Medial epicondylitis injection.

Physical therapy that focuses on gentle stretching and strengthening should also be used. In the acute phase, modalities such as ultrasound and soft tissue mobilization can be employed.

Aggressive conservative treatment is very successful for this condition with >85% making a full recovery. When necessary, surgical treatment involves epicondylar debridement. If the ulnar nerve is found to be involved, it can be decompressed at the time of surgery.

MEDIAL EPICONDYLITIS INJECTION

After informed consent is obtained, identify the medial epicondyle.

The authors favor using a 25-gauge, 1.5 inch needle, 20 mg of triamcinolone acetate and 1 cc of 1% lidocaine. Mark the point of maximal tenderness over the distal to the medial epicondyle.

Sterilize this area using iodine swabs x 3 and an alcohol pad. Using sterile technique, aim the needle perpendicular into the point of maximal tenderness. Always aspirate before injecting. If blood is found in the aspirate, reposition. There should be no aspirate in this injection. If resistance is felt, do not inject. Resistance could indicate that the needle is in the tendon. Never inject directly into the tendon. Reposition and aspirate again. When there is no aspirate and the injectate flows smoothly, inject. Clean the iodine off with alcohol pads. Note that some physicians favor using 40 mg of triamcinolone acetate. In the authors' experience, 20 mg is sufficient.

CUBITAL TUNNEL SYNDROME

Background

Compression of the ulnar nerve in the elbow (cubital tunnel syndrome) is the second most common peripheral nerve entrapment syndrome (the most common is carpal tunnel syndrome). The ulnar nerve is typically compressed as it passes in the cubital tunnel, which is the groove on the posterior aspect of the medial epicondyle. This area is also sometimes called the "funny bone" because people strike it on the table by accident and feel tingling sensations in their elbow and hand. Another common location for entrapment of the ulnar nerve is between the humeral and ulnar heads of the flexor carpi ulnaris.

Clinical Presentation

Patients typically report gradual onset of achy medial elbow pain and numbness and tingling in the fourth and fifth digits. Less commonly, numbness and tingling may radiate more proximally into the upper arm. As the pathology progresses, patients may complain of a weak grip that manifests in difficulties performing certain activities of daily living such as opening jars.

Occasionally, patients identify a traumatic event that immediately precipitated symptoms. In this less common instance, the onset is not slow and progressive but rather sudden.

Physical Examination

A Tinel sign typically is present over the cubital tunnel that reproduces the patient's symptoms. This is a sensitive but not very specific finding (may have many false positives). The ulnar groove in the cubital tunnel can be palpated as the elbow is slowly flexed and extended. If the ulnar nerve slips out of the groove with palpation, it may indicate ulnar irritation in the groove.

Numbness may also be noted in the fourth and fifth digits.

Sustained maximal flexion of the elbow is a good test for cubital tunnel syndrome. If this reproduces the patient's symptoms of numbness and tingling within 1 minute of maximal flexion, the test is considered positive. If it takes >1 minute, the test is considered negative.

Intrinsic hand strength may be diminished. Test finger adduction and abduction. Be sure to compare intrinsic hand strength to the asymptomatic side because the weakness may be subtle, particularly in the earlier stages of the pathology.

The Froment sign is a good way to assess for ulnar nerve entrapment. This sign specifically tests for strength in the adductor pollicis. The patient is asked to hold a piece of paper between his extended thumb and flat palm while the physician tries to pull the piece of paper away. In a patient with ulnar nerve palsy and adductor pollicis weakness, the patient flexes the flexor pollicis longus of the thumb to maintain hold of the paper.

Diagnostic Studies

EMG/NCV studies may be performed to establish the diagnosis. Although not typical, if only sensory nerve fibers are involved in the cubital tunnel syndrome, the study may result in a false-negative result.

Treatment

Activity modification to limit elbow flexion and keep direct pressure off the cubital tunnel is first-line treatment. A lightweight plastic arm splint or sports elbow protector can be worn at night to limit movement and decrease nocturnal irritation. Ice can be helpful. Physical or occupational therapy that teaches the patient how to avoid putting stress on the ulnar nerve as it passes through the cubital tunnel, along with stretching and strengthening exercises, should be considered.

Because this is not an inflammatory process, corticosteroid injection around the nerve is not recommended.

If symptoms persist despite aggressive conservative care for >3 months, or if symptoms are particularly severe and/or weakness is progressive, surgical decompression and transposition of the ulnar nerve is an option.

ULNAR COLLATERAL LIGAMENT INJURY

Background

The ulnar collateral ligament (UCL) is one of the primary elbow stabilizers. Young athletes who participate in repetitive throwing sports (e.g., baseball) are particularly prone to injury because of the repeated valgus stresses placed on the ligament that can lead to inflammation, microtears, and rupture.

Clinical Presentation

Patients are typically younger and report gradually increasing medial elbow pain that is worse with overhead throwing. Rest and ice generally make the pain better. Patients may reveal having thrown an excessive number of pitches. Patients also might report a similar pain in past seasons that went away when the season ended.

In patients with a rupture (which is relatively rare), patients may report a sudden popping sensation and intense pain in their medial elbow that occurred while throwing.

Physical Examination

Tenderness is typically noted over the UCL. There may be pain and/or slight loss of range of motion with full elbow extension. Ecchymosis and swelling is generally not present unless a frank rupture occurred. Valgus stressing of the elbow may elicit pain and, less commonly, reveal increased joint opening. The normal side should always be compared with the injured side.

Diagnostic Studies

Radiographs should be obtained and may reveal bony abnormalities. Magnetic resonance imaging with intra-articular contrast is the diagnostic imaging of choice. However, it should be noted that potential dye leakage in a chronic injury may have false-negative results.

Treatment

Protection, restricted activity, ice, compression, elevation (PRICE), judicious use of NSAIDs, and physical therapy that focuses on range of motion and strengthening exercises are first-line treatment. Steroid injections are not recommended for this disorder and may actually worsen the condition. If symptoms persist despite conservative care, surgical reconstruction may be considered. If surgery is undergone, postoperative rehabilitation may take at least 1 year.

Prior to return-to-sport, the patient should undergo a progressive throwing therapy program as well as strengthening of the surrounding musculature.

For prevention of the injury, it is crucial that young athletes not overstress their elbow by throwing too many pitches. The guidelines of the 2007 Little League board of directors state that youths 17 and 18 years of age should have a maximum pitch count of 105 per day. Youths 13 to 16 years should have a maximum pitch count of 95 per day. Youths 11 and 12 years of age should have a maximum pitch count of 85 per day, and youths ≤10 years should have a maximum pitch count of 75 per day. In addition, for youths ≤16 years, if they have ≥61 pitches, they need a minimum of 3 days of rest. If they have 41 to 60 pitches, they need 2 days minimum of rest; 21 to 40 pitches require at least 1 day of rest. For pitchers 17 and 18 years of age, if they have ≥76 pitches, they require at least 3 days of rest, 51 to 75 pitches require at least 2 days of rest, and 26 to 50 require at least 1 day of rest.

OLECRANON BURSITIS

Background

The olecranon bursa is very superficial and the elbows are often in contact with hard surfaces. This combination makes olecranon bursitis from prolonged irritation (leaning on one's elbows) or sudden trauma (falling onto the elbow) a relatively common cause of posterior elbow pain. The bursa can also become infected. Septic olecranon bursitis is less common, but it is important that it not be missed because prompt treatment is important to prevent potential spreading of the infection.

Clinical Presentation

Patients typically report gradual onset of focal posterior elbow pain. If a distinct trauma was involved, or if precipitated by an infection, the pain develops suddenly. The pain may be quite intense and limit full range of motion. Pressure exacerbates the pain. Patients also note swelling of the elbow.

Physical Examination

Patients typically have a posterior elbow swelling that is clearly demarcated and tender to the touch. If the bursa is erythematous and swollen, infection should be suspected. Likewise, if the patient has a fever, infection should be suspected.

Diagnostic Studies

If infection or crystalline deposit (gout or pseudogout) is at all suspected, the bursa should be aspirated and sent for Gram stain, culture, cell count, and crystal analysis. Normal white blood cell (WBC) count is <200/mL. A WBC of 200 to 2,000/mL is considered noninflammatory. A WBC of 2,000 to 100,000/mL is considered inflammatory. WBC >100,000/mL indicates sepsis.

If infection is suspected, lab work also may be sent to evaluate the complete blood count with WBC differential. If rheumatoid arthritis is suspected, rheumatoid factor and erythrocyte sedimentation rate may be sent.

If a trauma precipitated symptoms, radiographs may be obtained to rule out fracture.

Treatment

If the bursal effusion is large, it should be aspirated and sent for analysis as described earlier if the fluid looks at all suspicious. This aspiration may be therapeutic as well as diagnostic. Note that if the aspirate appears septic, or if sepsis is suspected, the patient may be started on empirical antibiotics. The patient should then be treated with activity modification, ice, and NSAIDs for 1 week. Elbow pads can also be used to cushion the elbows during everyday activities while the inflammation calms down.

If the patient is still symptomatic 1 week later, he or she returns to the physician. If Gram stain and cultures of the fluid are negative, the bursa is aspirated again. If the fluid remains aseptic, an injection of corticosteroid and lidocaine into the bursa can be very therapeutic. The patient can then also use a compressive neoprene or elastic elbow sleeve to help keep the bursal fluid from reaccumulating.

If the bursal effusion is small and only minimally bothersome, the patient may be treated with activity modification, ice, and NSAIDs alone. If the symptoms worsen or persist, aspiration may be appropriate.

If the olecranon bursitis is found to be septic, the patient should immediately be started on organism-specific antibiotics based on the culture and sensitivity of the aspirate. Depending on the organism and the immunity status of the individual, intravenous antibiotics in the hospital may be necessary. Surgical decompression or daily bursal aspiration should be performed.

PRONATOR SYNDROME

Background

In pronator syndrome, the median nerve is compressed in the proximal forearm. Although the exact site of nerve injury is variable, compression between the two muscular heads in the pronator teres is common.

Clinical Presentation

Patients typically present with vague complaints of anterior (volar) forearm pain that is exacerbated by activity and improved with rest. Patients also may complain of easy fatigability of the forearm. Patients sometimes also complain of numbness in the distal median nerve distribution, including the first three digits and the radial side of the fourth digit. Occasionally, the pain may radiate into the upper arm.

Physical Examination

Tinel sign should be elicited by tapping over the site of entrapment, about 4 cm distal to the antebrachial crease.

In addition, if resisted pronation reproduces symptoms within 60 seconds, this is suggestive of pronator syndrome. Numbness may be found over the median nerve distribution distal to the site of compression. The thenar muscles may also be found to be weak and/or atrophied when compared with the asymptomatic side.

Diagnostic Studies

The EMG/NCV test is typically normal in patients with pronator syndrome. Radiographs may be obtained to rule out other pathology.

Treatment

Conservative care includes rest, ice, NSAIDs, activity modification, and physical therapy. A corticosteroid and anesthetic injection also may provide relief. If symptoms persist for >3 months, or if symptoms are particularly severe and/or progressive, surgical decompression may be performed.

ANTERIOR INTEROSSEOUS NERVE SYNDROME

Background

In the anterior interosseous nerve (AIN) syndrome, the median nerve passes the elbow just medial to the biceps tendon. About 4 to 6 cm distal to the elbow, the AIN branches. The AIN is a pure motor nerve and supplies the flexor pollicis longus, pronator quadratus, and flexor digitorum profundus to the second digit.

Clinical Presentation

Patients typically present complaining of vague pain in the forearm and weakness with their pinch grasp.

Physical Examination

The classic test is the OK sign. In this test, patients are asked to make the OK sign with their fingers. If they have AIN, they are unable to make the sign. Instead, their distal interphalangeal joint and first digit interphalangeal joint will hyperextend, forming more of a triangle (Figs. 3.6A and 3.6B).

Diagnostic Studies

EMG/NCS may be helpful to establish the diagnosis and rule out other potential etiologies.

Treatment

Conservative care includes rest, NSAIDs, and splinting. A short course of physical therapy may also be helpful. Surgical options include surgical exploration with decompression of the AIN.

ELBOW DISLOCATION

Background

Elbows are typically dislocated posteriorly unless associated with a fracture. The elbow is the third most commonly dislocated joint in the adult (behind shoulder and finger) and most common in pediatrics.

Clinical Presentation

Patients typically report a history of falling onto an outstretched hand that immediately precipitated pain, swelling, and an inability to bend the elbow.

Physical Examination

The dislocation is readily apparent to inspection and palpation. In a posterior dislocation, the olecranon is very prominent and the forearm appears shortened. A thorough neurovascular examination must be completed to rule out associated injury.

Diagnostic Studies

Radiographs are important to obtain to rule out associated fracture.

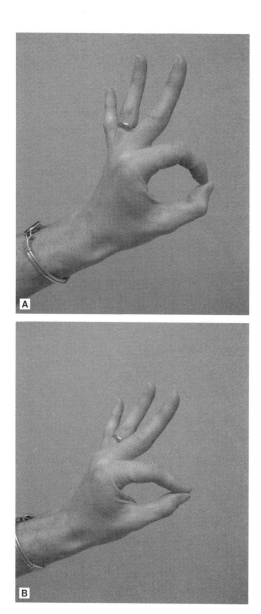

Figure 3.6 (A) OK sign normal. (B) OK sign abnormal (positive sign: anterior interosseous nerve syndrome).

Treatment

The dislocation should be reduced as soon as possible. Because of the possibility of neurovascular injury, the dislocation should be performed by an emergency department physician, orthopedic surgeon, or other musculoskeletal medicine specialist with experience in manual reductions. After reduction, the neurovascular status is rechecked and radiographs are obtained to confirm alignment.

Surgery may be necessary if there is any associated neurovascular compromise, the dislocation is nonreducible, or if there are any associated fractures.

ELBOW FRACTURES

Background

A radial fracture is the most common form of elbow fracture and results from a fall onto an outstretched arm.

An olecranon fracture typically results from a fall onto a semiflexed, supinated forearm or may occur after a direct blow to the olecranon.

Clinical Presentation

Patients typically present with a history of a fall that immediately precipitated pain, swelling, and possibly ecchymosis.

Patients with a radial head fracture have pain primarily on the lateral aspect of the elbow. Patients with an olecranon fracture have more posterior pain over the lateral aspect of the elbow.

Physical Examination

Inspection reveals swelling. Abrasions or deeper wounds may be present secondary to the trauma. Palpation helps determine if the fracture is displaced.

In a radial head fracture, the effusion may be over the lateral elbow. The radial head is tender to palpation. Passive elbow range of motion may be restricted by pain. The patient may be unable to pronate the forearm.

It is always critical to perform a neurovascular examination to ensure that the trauma did not result in further injury. In an olecranon fracture, the ulnar nerve is the one most commonly injured.

Diagnostic Studies

Radiographs are required to confirm the diagnosis and extent of fracture (Figs. 3.7A–C).

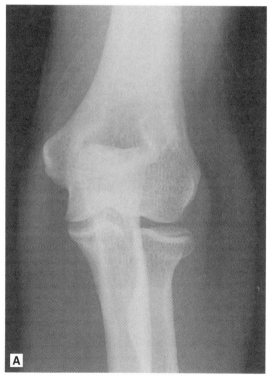

Figure 3.7 **(A)** Elbow fracture. Anteroposterior elbow radiograph shows a minimally impacted fracture of the articular surface of the radial head.

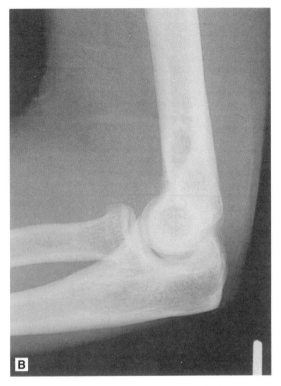

Figure 3.7 *(continued)*   **(B)** Lateral radiograph shows a triangular lucency in the soft tissues anterior to the distal humerus (anterior fat pad sign). The fracture is obliquely oriented and difficult to see.

Treatment

If a radial head fracture is present but nondisplaced, or minimally displaced, it may be treated with a sling or splint and transitioned to early range of motion exercises. If the fracture is displaced by ≥3 mm, angulated by >30%, involves 33% or more of the articular surface (rule of 3s), and/or is severely comminuted, surgery is preferable.

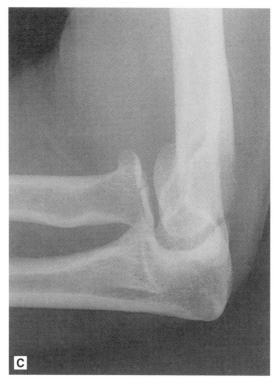

Figure 3.7 *(continued)*   **(C)** Oblique radiograph shows the fracture. (From Chew F, Roberts C. *Musculoskeletal Imaging: A Teaching File.* 2nd ed. Philadelphia, Pa: Lippincott Williams & Wilkins, 2006, with permission.)

If an olecranon fracture is present but nondisplaced, a posterior splint, with the elbow held in about 40 to 60 degrees of flexion, may be used. Some physicians immobilize at 90 degrees. The elbow should have a repeat radiograph in 1 week to ensure the fracture has not displaced. Depending on the extent of injury, range of motion exercises should begin at 2 to 3 weeks postinjury.

If the olecranon fracture is displaced >2 mm, surgical treatment is typically required.

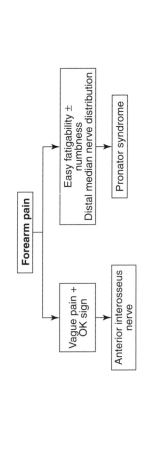

Forearm pain

Vague pain + OK sign

Anterior interosseus nerve

Easy fatigability ± numbness Distal median nerve distribution

Pronator syndrome

Wrist and Hand Pain

4

Red Flag Signs and Symptoms

Any of these signs and symptoms should prompt urgent evaluation and appropriate intervention:

Fevers
Chills
Hot, swollen joint
Progressive neurologic symptoms
Loss of pulses

CARPAL TUNNEL SYNDROME

Background

Carpal tunnel syndrome (CTS) is the most common compressive neuropathy. The carpal bones form the floor and walls of the tunnel, and the rigid flexor retinaculum attaches to the trapezium and scaphoid bones to form the rigid roof. Through this rigid tunnel pass the eight flexor tendons covered in a common sheath as well as the flexor pollicis longus tendon in its own sheath. The median nerve rests superficially just dorsal to the flexor retinaculum. Diabetes mellitus, thyroid dysfunction, pregnancy, rheumatoid arthritis, and other medical conditions predispose to the development of CTS.

Clinical Presentation

Patients typically present with achy pain and numbness that radiates from the wrist into the first three digits and radial side of the fourth digit. It is not unusual for patients frequently to complain of pain and numbness in

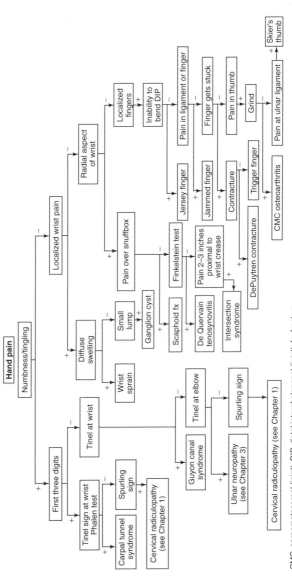

CMC, carpometacarpal (joint); DIP, distal interphalangeal (joint); fx, fracture.

the whole hand. Patients may report waking up in the middle of the night with increased symptoms and then shaking the hand to "wake it up," "get the blood flowing," and decrease the pain and numbness. Symptoms may be exacerbated during activities such as typing or knitting. In general, activities that require repetitive wrist flexion (typing in a suboptimal anatomic position) or repetitive wrist extension exacerbate symptoms.

As the syndrome progresses, symptoms may become more constant. Patients may also note weakness in their grip, including difficulty with activities such as opening jars or buttoning a shirt. They may also report dropping things. Sometimes they perceive this weakness as "clumsiness" in their hands.

Physical Examination

The three classic tests for CTS are the Tinel sign, Phalen test, and carpal compression test. A positive Tinel sign (Fig. 4.1) occurs when repetitive tapping over the median nerve as it

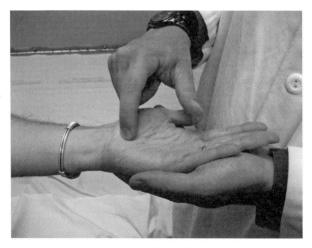

Figure 4.1   Tinel sign for carpal tunnel syndrome.

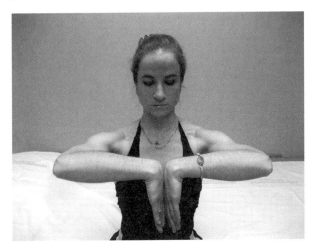

Figure 4.2   Phalen test.

passes through the carpal tunnel elicits symptoms in the median nerve distribution. In the Phalen test (Fig. 4.2), the patient places both wrists in full flexion and juxtaposes the dorsal aspect of each hand against the other. If symptoms are reproduced within 1 minute, the test is positive for CTS. Symptoms typically occur in the first 10 to 20 seconds if the patient has CTS.

In the carpal compression test (Fig. 4.3), the physician places steady, firm pressure over the carpal tunnel. If symptoms are reproduced in 30 seconds, the test is considered indicative of CTS.

Patients may report numbness to light palpation over the median nerve distribution in the hand. The thenar eminence should *not* be numb because the cutaneous branch of the median nerve supplies this region and it branches prior to the carpal tunnel.

In more advanced cases, patients may have wasting of the thenar eminence and/or thenar weakness, which manifests by the patient having difficulty opposing the thumb.

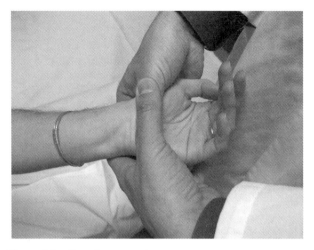

Figure 4.3   Carpal compression test.

Diagnostic Studies

An electromyelography/nerve conduction velocity (EMG/NCV) study is the study of choice to distinguish CTS from other pathologies such as a cervical radiculitis or ulnar neuropathy. EMG/NCS also is able to determine the severity of disease. Typically, symptoms correlate with amount of nerve damage. But occasionally a patient with moderate or even mild symptoms may have significant nerve damage when tested with EMG/NCS. This is important to note because it needs to be addressed more urgently or at least needs to be followed more closely. Once the motor nerves are significantly damaged, strength may take a long time to return or may not return. There is debate as to which patients with suspected CTS should receive an electrodiagnostic study. Certainly, any patient considering surgery would benefit from EMG/NCS. Some physicians believe that most, if not all, patients with CTS should receive EMG/NCS both to document the severity of disease and to note which patients need closer following and/or more aggressive intervention because of nerve damage.

Recent studies have shown that the use of ultrasound for the assessment of the median nerve may be a promising noninvasive imaging study. With the use of ultrasound the edema of the median nerve is assessed. EMG/NCS still remains the standard for diagnosing median nerve pathology.

Treatment

In mild cases a resting wrist splint used at night to keep the wrist in the neutral position may be sufficient. While sleeping, people have a tendency to flex their wrists, placing stress on the nerve in the tunnel. In the case of CTS, this may add constant irritation to the nerve and slow healing.

A short course of nonsteroidal anti-inflammatory drugs may also be helpful. In addition, patients should undergo a short course of occupational (or physical) therapy. In therapy, patients should work on ergonomics education, postural mechanics, strengthening exercises, and tendon gliding exercises. In the acute phase, ice can be used to help reduce inflammation. In addition, a workplace assessment (or education about workspace adjustments) is critical to ensure that repetitive stresses aren't being placed on the carpal tunnel daily.

If the symptoms are more constant and/or bothersome to the patient, an effective treatment is a steroid and anesthetic injection into the carpal tunnel (Fig. 4.4), which may speed recovery. Ultrasound guidance may help with injection accuracy.

CARPAL TUNNEL INJECTION

After informed consent is obtained, identify the carpal tunnel. The authors favor using a 25-gauge, 1.5 inch needle, 40 mg of triamcinolone acetate, and 1 mL of 1% lidocaine. Mark a spot in the middle of the proximal wrist crease. Sterilize this area using three iodine swabs and an alcohol pad. Using sterile technique, aim the needle at a 45-degree angle to the tunnel and inject distally. Always aspirate before injecting. If blood is found in the aspirate, reposition. There should be no aspirate in this injection. If resistance is felt, do not inject. Resistance could indicate that the needle is in a tendon. *Never inject directly into a tendon.* Reposition and aspirate again. When there is no aspirate and the injectate flows smoothly, inject. Clean the iodine off with alcohol pads.

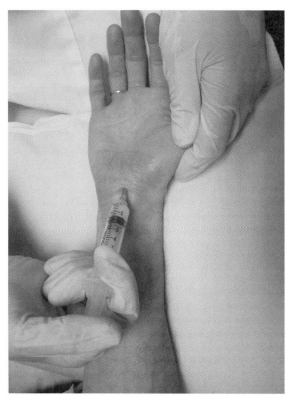

Figure 4.4   Carpal tunnel injection.

For more constant symptoms, the wrist splints can be used more frequently.

If conservative care is not effective, surgical release of the tunnel may be needed.

Of note, if a pregnant patient develops CTS, the symptoms may resolve spontaneously postpregnancy.

If a patient has an underlying untreated condition causing the CTS (e.g., hypothyroidism) it is of course critical to treat it. Treatment of the underlying condition may alleviate the CTS symptoms as well.

DE QUERVAIN TENOSYNOVITIS

Background

De Quervain tenosynovitis is an inflammation of the tendons in the first dorsal compartment of the wrist. These tendons are the abductor pollicis longus (APL) and extensor pollicis brevis (EPB). They can be remembered by the mnemonic "All peanut lovers (APL) eat peanut butter (EPB)." De Quervain tenosynovitis can be caused by repetitive microtrauma or, less commonly, a sudden trauma to the tendons.

Clinical Presentation

Patients complain of pain localized to the dorsolateral aspect of the wrist over the radial styloid. The pain is classically exacerbated by movements of the thumb. A detailed history often reveals the patient has begun a new activity that involves repetitive thumb use. For example, the patient may be a young mother who has been repetitively picking up her newborn. Other common causes include taking on a new hobby such as knitting, golf, computer use, or gardening. These activities exacerbate the pain. Sometimes, there is mild swelling over the painful area.

Physical Examination

Note any swelling over the first dorsal compartment of the wrist. The Finkelstein test should be performed. In this test, the patient makes a fist with his thumb fully flexed *under* his four fingers. The physician then passively applies an ulnar deviating force to the wrist. This test may be "positive" in many asymptomatic people. So it is important to ensure the test reproduces the patient's typical symptoms to consider the test positive. In addition, the asymptomatic side should be tested.

Diagnostic Studies

No imaging studies are routine for this condition. They should be ordered to rule out other pathologies (such as may be the case with an acute injury to the tendons precipitating symptoms to rule out fracture).

Treatment

Initial treatment consists of the patient using a thumb spica splint. This splint immobilizes the thumb and wrist. Ice may also be used as an excellent anti-inflammatory agent in this area. The patient may benefit from a short course of occupational therapy.

If symptoms are severe or the patient's symptoms persist despite 2 to 3 weeks of more conservative therapy, an injection into the tendon sheath may be performed (Fig. 4.5). As always, it is important not to inject directly into the tendon itself. Ultrasound can be used to help with visualization of the injection. In addition to the usual risks of injection (e.g., infection, bleeding, allergic reaction, tendon weakening, transient elevation of blood glucose), because of the location of the injection there is a risk of skin hypopigmentation (related to the superficiality of the injection). Subcutaneous atrophy has been reported to (very rarely) extend through the lymphatics more proximally in the forearm and cause injury to the radial sensory nerve. Injury to the radial sensory nerve may result in anesthesia over the first web space of the dorsal hand and dorsal thumb. This generally resolves within a few hours. Rarely, if the radial nerve is severely injured by direct needle penetration, persistent pain may result in the superficial radial nerve distribution.

In severe recalcitrant cases, surgical decompression of the first dorsal compartment may be necessary.

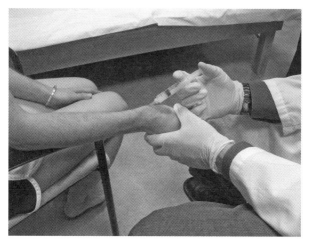

Figure 4.5   De Quervain injection.

DE QUERVAIN TENOSYNOVITIS INJECTION

After informed consent is obtained, identify the point of maximal tenderness along the tendon sheath of the abductor pollicis longus and extensor pollicis brevis. The authors favor using a 25-gauge, 1.5 inch needle, 20 mg of triamcinolone acetate, and 1 mL of 1% lidocaine. Mark a spot approximately 3 cm distal to the point of maximal tenderness. Sterilize this area using three iodine swabs and an alcohol pad. Using sterile technique, aim the needle at a 30-degree angle to the tendon and inject proximally. Always aspirate before injecting. If blood is found in the aspirate, reposition. There should be no aspirate in this injection. If resistance is felt, do not inject. Resistance could indicate that the needle is in the tendon. *Never inject directly into a tendon.* Reposition and aspirate again. When there is no aspirate and the injectate flows smoothly, inject. Clean the iodine off with alcohol pads.

FIRST CARPOMETACARPAL JOINT ARTHRITIS (BASE OF THUMB ARTHRITIS)

Background

The first carpometacarpal (CMC) is the hand joint most commonly affected by osteoarthritis. It is an idiopathic condition that occurs primarily in women older than 40 years. Rheumatoid arthritis may also affect this joint (although there are usually systemic symptoms and bilateral involvement of the joints).

Clinical Presentation

Patients complain of pain at the base of their thumb that is exacerbated by pinching. Patients may complain of "weakness" in their pinch and grip strength. Patients may also describe stiffness in their thumb. Less commonly, patients report that the thumb clicks and grinds with certain movements.

Physical Examination

Patients typically have tenderness over the dorsal and radial aspect of the thumb. The hallmark of the condition is a positive grind test (Fig. 4.6). In this test, the physician grips the patient's proximal phalanx and grinds it into the trapezium (carpal bone). When this maneuver reproduces the patient's symptoms, it is considered positive. Crepitus and/or instability may also be noted with the maneuver.

Diagnostic Studies

Radiographs reveal joint space narrowing, sclerosis, cystic changes, and other signs of osteoarthritis. Of note, many asymptomatic people may have radiographic changes consistent with CMC osteoarthritis. Therefore, the radiographs are used to confirm clinical suspicion but are not diagnostic in and of themselves.

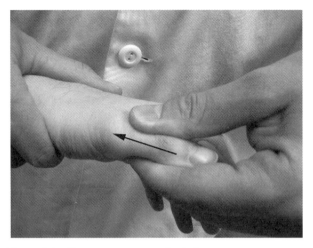

Figure 4.6   First carpometacarpal grind test.

When the diagnosis is in question, a diagnostic intra-articular injection of anesthetic can be performed. If this alleviates the symptoms, it confirms the diagnosis. If corticosteroid is added to the injectate, the injection can be therapeutic as well.

Treatment

Conservative care includes occupational therapy to improve pain and function by stretching and strengthening. Modalities such as paraffin and heat can be useful in occupational therapy. Topical analgesic creams are helpful. Some physicians commonly place the thumb in a spica splint for a period of 2 to 3 weeks to immobilize the thumb and let the acute inflammatory phase calm down.

An injection of corticosteroid and anesthetic into the joint (Fig. 4.7) may also be very helpful. These injections may provide ≥3 months of relief when successful.

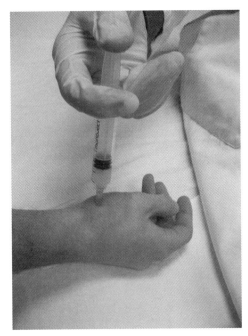

Figure 4.7   First carpometacarpal injection.

FIRST CARPOMETACARPAL INJECTION

After informed consent is obtained, identify the first CMC joint. The authors favor using a 25-gauge, 1.5 inch needle, 20 mg of triamcinolone acetate, and 1 mL of 1% lidocaine. Mark the CMC joint. Sterilize this area using three iodine swabs and an alcohol pad. Using sterile technique, aim the needle perpendicular to the joint. Always aspirate before injecting. If blood is found in the aspirate, reposition. There should be no aspirate in this injection. If resistance is felt, do not inject. Resistance may mean you are not in the joint. Reposition and aspirate again. When there is no aspirate and the injectate flows smoothly, inject. Clean the iodine off with alcohol pads.

When conservative care is no longer effective, surgical options such as joint fusion, ligament reconstruction, and tendon interposition (when there is instability of the joint) with partial or total trapezium resection may be required.

SKIER'S THUMB (GAMEKEEPER'S THUMB)

Background

Skier's thumb is an injury of the ulnar collateral ligament (UCL) of the thumb. When the injury occurs as a result of skiing, it typically happens after an injury in which the pole places an abducting force onto the UCL during a fall. The injury is also called gamekeeper's thumb. Gamekeeper's thumb was originally described in 1955 in 24 Scottish gamekeepers who experienced UCL laxity after repetitively sacrificing small game (e.g., rabbits, chickens) by breaking their necks between their thumb and index fingers and the ground. The injury may be a result of sudden trauma. Patients typically describe a trauma to the inside of their thumb over the UCL. The trauma may have been a skiing accident, rugby tackle, fall onto an outstretched arm, or any other injury that forcefully abducts the thumb. The injury may also result from repetitive abduction or hyperextension of the thumb. This is seen in hockey players who repetitively jam their thumb into the hockey stick.

Clinical Presentation

The patient usually presents complaining of pain localized to the medial aspect of the thumb. Depending on the mechanism of injury, the pain may be acute as seen in traumatic events or of gradual onset that is typical of repetitive trauma. Complaints of weakness with grip strength because of pain are also common.

Physical Examination

Tenderness and swelling may be present on the ulnar aspect of the MCP joint. In the case of an acute injury, ecchymosis may be present.

If fracture is suspected, radiographs should be obtained prior to the following examination maneuver. Once the fracture is ruled out, the forearm is placed midway between pronation and supination in neutral position. The physician then stabilizes the patient's first metacarpal with one hand and applies a gradual radial stress on the thumb, stressing the UCL (Fig. 4.8). If there is excessive glide, this is indicative of a UCL injury. Comparison with the asymptomatic side is important. If the testing is too painful, a local anesthetic can be injected.

Diagnostic Studies

Radiographs may be obtained to rule out fracture and/or avulsion injury. If surgery is being contemplated, ultrasound can be obtained, but magnetic resonance imaging (MRI) has greater sensitivity and specificity.

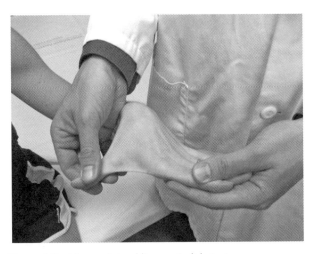

Figure 4.8 Ulnar collateral ligament glide test.

Treatment

If the ligament is loosened but not ruptured, conservative care with immobilization may be used. Immobilization may last from 3 to 6 weeks depending on the lesion and recovery speed. Immobilization is typically followed by use of a thumb spica for an additional 2 to 4 weeks and rehabilitation therapy. If a full rupture is present, the lesion is called a Stener lesion, and surgical repair is needed or the MCP may never regain full stability.

TRIGGER FINGER

Background

Trigger finger, also called stenosing tenosynovitis, is caused by a thickening of the flexor tendon or first annular pulley. As the tendon slides back and forth during flexion, it moves through a series of pulleys. When the tendon or pulley is inflamed, it becomes thickened. The tendon then gets caught on the pulley and the finger locks. When it is forced through the pulley, the tendon glides easily. This is why trigger finger "triggers." The finger gets stuck and then releases and glides easily throughout the rest of its range of motion. Trigger finger may be associated with rheumatoid arthritis or diabetes, but it often is idiopathic, occurring most often in patients older than 40 years.

Clinical Presentation

Patients typically report that their finger "catches," "locks," "gets stuck," or "triggers." Pain associated with the triggering may or sometimes may not be present. When pain is present, it typically occurs over the proximal interphalangeal (PIP) or metacarpophalangeal (MCP) joint. Any digit, or multiple digits, may be afflicted. Sometimes patients awaken with their finger "locked" and have to slowly unlock it. Patients with diabetes or rheumatoid arthritis are more likely to have multiple digit involvement.

Physical Examination

On examination, the involved digit becomes fixed in a flexed position. The patient then typically forces the digit into extension or uses other digits to help the involved digit unlock. As the digit unlocks, it "triggers" and moves through the restriction. This may or may not elicit pain from the patient.

At the distal palmar crease, overlying the MCP joint, a tender nodule is typically palpable. Occasionally, the nodule may be palpated more distally over the PIP.

Diagnostic Studies

None are routinely necessary.

Treatment

The cornerstone of treatment is an injection into the tendon sheath, or palpable nodule, at the site of maximal tenderness (Fig. 4.9). Care should be taken not to inject into the tendon. Ultrasound may be useful to guide injection accuracy. This injection is typically very effective for trigger finger.

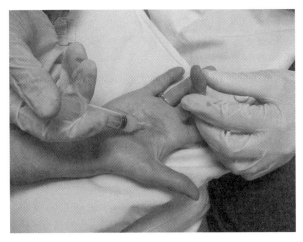

Figure 4.9   Trigger finger injection.

TRIGGER FINGER INJECTION

After informed consent is obtained, identify the nodule causing the trigger. (Others inject from a distal starting point.) The authors favor using a 25- or 30-gauge needle, 20 mg of triamcinolone acetate, and 0.5 mL of 1% lidocaine. Mark the spot over the nodule responsible for the triggering. Sterilize this area using three iodine swabs and an alcohol pad. Using sterile technique, aim the needle at a 45-degree angle to the nodule and inject. The angle can be from the proximal or distal direction. The authors typically favor a proximal position in which the needle is angled distally. Always aspirate before injecting. If blood is found in the aspirate, reposition. There should be no aspirate in this injection. If resistance is felt, do not inject. Reposition and aspirate again. When there is no aspirate and the injectate flows smoothly, inject. Clean the iodine off with alcohol pads.

Some physicians also give a splint for the involved finger to keep it extended during much of the day and/or night for a week after injection.

If symptoms persist, the injection may be repeated after 3 to 4 weeks. A third injection may also be performed if symptoms are alleviated but then later recur. Care must be taken with multiple injections because they increase the risk of tendon rupture. The digital sensory nerve also can occasionally be injured.

If symptoms persist despite injection(s), surgical release may be indicated.

GANGLION CYST

Background

Ganglion cysts are common and can occur in any synovial joint or sheath. A ganglion cyst is simply a break in the capsule of a joint or tendon synovial sheath that results in an outpouching of contained synovial fluid. Cysts can be single or multilobulated. In the wrist and hand, they most commonly occur in women from 20 to 70 years of age. However, they may occur at any age, in both men and women. They are idiopathic and often disappear spontaneously.

Clinical Presentation

Patients often present with an asymptomatic swelling or "lump" on the dorsal aspect of their wrist. If pain is present, it is typically "achy" and associated with wrist movements. If the ganglion is pressing on the median or ulnar nerve, symptoms may radiate in the distribution of the nerve. Other common locations for the cyst include the palmar surface of the wrist and the flexor tendon sheath of the digits. When a cyst is present in the distal interphalangeal joint (DIP), it is a mucous cyst.

Physical Examination

The ganglion is well circumscribed and smooth to palpation. The most common position for the ganglion on the dorsal wrist is over the scapholunate joint. There may be some mild tenderness to palpation. Shining a penlight at the ganglion transilluminates it. If the mass is not translucent, it is likely a solid tumor. A bluish discoloration of the mass raises suspicion that the mass is vascular.

A ganglion on the palmar surface of the wrist may be more difficult to appreciate. These ganglia may extend beneath the radial artery and thus feel pulsatile. Imaging may be required to identify these masses further.

Diagnostic Studies

Radiographs may be obtained to rule out bony pathology, but they are not always necessary. If the diagnosis is in doubt (such as with a palmar wrist ganglion), MRI may be needed. Ultrasound also may be helpful for this purpose.

Treatment

Because most ganglia in the wrist are asymptomatic or only mildly symptomatic, and most resolve spontaneously, education may be all that is needed. If the patient is having bothersome symptoms, including being disturbed by the cosmetic deformity, nonsurgical options include aspiration of the cyst. Unfortunately, aspiration results in about a 90% recurrence rate. When aspiration is unsuccessful, surgical excision may be required. Postsurgery, recurrence rates are <10%. Aspiration can be done with ultrasound guidance, particularly on if the cyst is on the palmar surface of the wrist where there is a risk of radial artery injury with aspiration (for this reason, too, surgery is perhaps a better initial treatment when the cyst is on the palmar surface).

A ganglion in the flexor tendon sheath can also be treated with aspiration and/or rupture of the cyst with local anesthetic. Injections in the flexor tendon sheath, particularly when the purpose is to rupture the cyst, must be done with great caution because of the proximity of the neurovascular bundle.

Caution must be taken with steroid injections into or near the superficial structures of the hand because of the risks of infection, skin and fat atrophy, and hypopigmentation.

Cysts in or around the DIP and/or fingernail should be treated surgically by a hand specialist because of the risk of infection. These cysts often coexist with Heberden nodes (osteophytes at the DIP), and these may be an underlying contributing factor. These osteophytes may be removed during surgery. Occasionally, a hand surgeon may attempt an anesthetic and corticosteroid injection into the cyst instead of surgery, but this should be done only by a specialist because of the complication risk.

JERSEY FINGER

Background

Jersey finger is a sprain, rupture, and/or avulsion of the flexor digitorum profundus (FDP). The FDP is responsible for flexing the DIP. Jersey finger typically results from an athlete reaching out to grab another athlete and getting his or her finger stuck in the opponent's jersey (commonly in football, ice hockey, rugby, etc.). The fourth digit is the finger most commonly affected because that is the digit most exposed when making a fist. Jersey finger can also result from a gradual erosion of the tendon in rheumatoid arthritis and other inflammatory arthritis conditions.

Clinical Presentation

Patients typically present with pain when moving the involved finger and an inability to bend at the DIP. Patients may initially think the injury is a "jammed finger" and so not seek care for several days. In patients with gradual erosion of the tendon, the patient may complain of noticing an inability to bend their DIP but no pain.

Physical Examination

On examination, the patient is able to flex the PIP but not the DIP. To test flexion of the DIP, hold the PIP in extension and have the patient flex the DIP. Tenderness and swelling may be present over the DIP. Also test sensation, which may be compromised in the distal digit if the digital nerves have been injured.

Diagnostic Studies

Radiographs should be obtained to evaluate for avulsion and/or other fracture.

Treatment

Surgical repair of the injury is typically required and should be done within a few days of injury if possible. After surgical correction, patients may benefit from a course of therapy to strengthen the surrounding muscles and improve proprioception in the injured area to help prevent repeat injury.

SCAPHOID FRACTURE

Background

Scaphoid fractures are particularly important wrist fractures for three reasons. First, they are the most common carpal fracture. Second, they are often misdiagnosed initially and thought to be only a "wrist sprain." Third, and most important, because of the poor vascular supply to the scaphoid (only the distal third receives significant blood flow), failure to recognize the lesion and provide appropriate care results in a relatively high rate of nonunion and osteonecrosis.

Clinical Presentation

Patients typically report a fall onto an outstretched hand that precipitated symptoms. Symptoms include pain and often swelling over the back and radial side of the wrist. Movement of the wrist typically exacerbates the pain.

Physical Examination

The hallmark physical examination finding of scaphoid fracture is pain over the anatomic snuffbox. Not all patients with pain in the anatomic snuffbox have a scaphoid fracture (many only have ligamentous damage), but many physicians believe that pain in this area should be treated as a scaphoid fracture until proven otherwise by imaging.

Diagnostic Studies

Radiographs should be obtained. However, if the initial radiographs are negative but clinical suspicion is present, the patient should be treated as if he or she has a scaphoid fracture because the fracture may not initially be evident radiographically. The radiographs should be repeated in 2 weeks. If they are still negative in 2 weeks, an MRI or bone scan may be obtained. If the patient requires an immediate definitive diagnosis (because of a need to return to sport or other activity), a bone scan may be performed 24 hours postinjury for definitive assessment (although this does not provide 100% sensitivity either). Computed tomography scan may be a good alternative to obtain 10 days postinjury.

Treatment

If snuffbox tenderness is present and significant, the patient should be treated as though he or she has a scaphoid fracture regardless of the initial radiographic result. Referral to a hand specialist is appropriate. The patient's thumb should be immobilized (a thumb spica splint is one option) and repeat radiographs or MRI scheduled. There is debate about optimal treatment for nondisplaced fractures, including how much of the lower arm should be casted. Surgical indications are also somewhat controversial. At the least, a scaphoid fracture needs close follow-up from a hand surgeon to monitor progress with nonsurgical care and/or discuss surgical options.

WRIST SPRAIN

Background

A wrist sprain is a relatively common injury to sustain after a fall onto an outstretched hand. Many ligaments in the wrist can be sprained. A sprain can occur on the radial (e.g., scapholunate ligament) or ulnar (e.g., triangular fibrocartilage complex injury) side. The diagnosis is primarily one of exclusion unless instability is noted. This is because it is most important to rule out other pathologies such as a fracture.

Clinical Presentation

Patients typically present with wrist pain after suffering a fall or other trauma to the wrist. Moving the wrist may exacerbate symptoms. A thorough neurovascular examination as well as strength and sensation testing should always be performed. If tenderness is elicited over the snuffbox, a scaphoid fracture should be suspected (see "Scaphoid Fracture" section).

Physical Examination

The involved area is characteristically tender. Swelling and/ or ecchymosis is occasionally present. Range of motion may be limited secondary to pain. Pain with resisted manual muscle testing also reveals the severity of the sprain. Palpation over the carpal bones, especially over the anatomic snuffbox, should be performed to determine the presence of a fracture.

Diagnostic Studies

Radiographs are typically obtained to rule out a fracture (e.g., distal radial fracture). If a specific injury is suspected such as a scaphoid fracture, additional imaging may be required.

Treatment

Protection, restricted activity, ice, compression, elevation (PRICE) is first-line therapy. If symptoms are significant, a Velcro wrist splint or plastic cast may be useful until symptoms improve. If a third-degree sprain is present, the patient may have instability of the wrist and a hand surgeon should be consulted.

INTERSECTION SYNDROME

Background

Intersection syndrome is a tenosynovitis of the second dorsal wrist tunnel. These are the extensor carpi radialis longus (ECRL) and extensor carpi radialis brevis (ECRB). This syndrome is much less common than De Quervain disease and is often confused with it. It is called "intersection syndrome" because the site of pathology is at the intersection of the first and second dorsal wrist compartments. Because of this, De Quervain disease and intersection syndrome may sometimes coexist.

Clinical Presentation

Patients complain of pain 2 to 3 inches proximal to the wrist crease on the radial side. Pain may be exacerbated with wrist movements. Often, patients report having started a new activity requiring repetitive wrist movements, particularly wrist flexion and extension, such as raking, gardening, or playing racket sports. The Finkelstein test may be positive.

Diagnostic Studies

None are routinely indicated.

Treatment

Treatment is similar to De Quervain disease. Initial treatment consists of activity modification alone and icing if the symptoms are very mild.

If symptoms are more significant, immobilization is used. The patient can use a cock-up wrist splint at 20 degrees of extension. A thumb spica splint (especially if De Quervain is also present) can also be used.

A short course of occupational therapy that focuses on strengthening and tendon stretching should be undergone once the patient is able to tolerate it.

A corticosteroid injection can be very effective in helping speed recovery.

Conservative care is typically very effective. In the rare instance when it is not, surgical decompression may be pursued.

JAMMED FINGER (FINGER SPRAIN)

Background

Finger sprain is a relatively common injury and occurs at collateral and/or volar capsular ligaments.

Clinical Presentation

Patients typically report having "jammed" their finger and subsequently experienced pain. Patients sometimes note swelling.

Physical Examination

Tenderness is noted over the involved ligament. If the MCP ulnar ligament is involved, the patient must be evaluated for possible skier's thumb (see section on skier's thumb for more details).

If the finger is deformed or if a fracture is suspected for any reason, radiographs should be ordered to rule out fracture prior to any stress testing of the fingers. The integrity of the ligament can be evaluated by gently stressing it to see if there is any instability. If there is increased angulation on one finger compared with its asymptomatic counterpart on the other hand, a third-degree sprain (complete tear) may be present.

Diagnostic Studies

Radiographs should be obtained to rule out fracture.

Treatment

If the ulnar ligament of the MCP joint is involved, see the "Skier's Thumb" section for diagnostic and treatment guidelines.

If it is a first- or second-degree sprain with no concomitant fracture or instability, nonsurgical care is very effective.

PRICE should be used. Taping the injured finger to the adjacent finger (buddy taping) can be used. The average healing time is about 2 to 6 weeks for a first-degree sprain and 8 to 14 weeks for a second-degree sprain.

If a third-degree sprain is present or there is instability, the patient may require surgical stabilization.

GUYON CANAL SYNDROME (ULNAR ENTRAPMENT AT THE WRIST)

Background

Guyon canal is a tunnel in the wrist through which the ulnar nerve passes. Guyon canal is formed by the pisiform and hamate bones and their connecting ligament. Causes include a space-occupying lesion (e.g., lipoma, ganglion, osteophyte) or repetitive trauma (e.g., repetitive heavy gripping, hammering, cycling).

Clinical Presentation

Patients typically have numbness and tingling (or "pins and needles") in the fifth and ulnar side of the fourth digit. Symptoms are sometimes worse in the morning and exacerbated with repetitive trauma (e.g., continued cycling, hammering, etc.). Patients sometimes complain of "weakness" or "clumsiness" in their hand. This may be due to decreased sensation. In some cases, the sensory fibers are spared and only the motor fibers are involved, in which case only weakness is present.

Physical Examination

Patients may have a positive Tinel sign over the canal. Sensation may be diminished over the palmar aspect of the fifth digit and ulnar side of the fourth digit. The dorsal aspect of the fourth and fifth digits should be normal because the sensory branch to this area branches prior to the canal.

Weakness may be noted with finger abduction. In advanced cases, atrophy may be noted of the hypothenar eminence.

Diagnostic Studies

EMG/NCV studies are very helpful to confirm the diagnosis and rule out other nerve involvement or other site of entrapment of the ulnar nerve (e.g., cubital tunnel syndrome).

Treatment

If repetitive trauma (e.g., hammering, working with the wrist bent down) is the cause of the symptoms, activity modification and occupational or physical therapy to work on body biomechanics and ergonomics is the treatment of choice.

If a space-occupying lesion is the cause, treatment is surgical to decompress the nerve.

DUPUYTREN DISEASE (VIKING DISEASE)

Background

Dupuytren disease is an abnormal thickening and contraction of the palmar fascia within the hand, possibly ultimately resulting in a fixed flexion contracture of the MCP and PIP joints. The disease is most common in men older than 40 years of Northern European descent. The fourth and fifth digits are the most commonly involved.

Clinical Presentation

Patients typically present with a history of progressive loss of ability to extend the MCP and PIP of the affected finger. Any digit may be involved, but the fourth is the most common. Patients may recall having a nodule in their distal palmar crease that was initially painful but then hardened and resolved. In some patients, the nodule persists and, rarely, continues to be painful. If the disease is more advanced, the patient may report difficulty with activities of daily living such as putting on gloves.

Physical Examination

Typical physical examination findings include a nodule in the distal aspect of the palm that is not tender to palpation (unless early in the disease). The thickening may extend along the tendon sheath into the PIP. Active and passive extension is limited in the MCP and sometimes the PIP. Within the available range of motion, strength is within normal limits. Sensation is intact.

Diagnostic Studies

None are routinely ordered.

Treatment

A patient with mild disease can initially be treated conservatively with nighttime splints and occupational therapy. Some physicians advocate use of an intralesional corticosteroid injection during the early stages of the disease.

Surgical intervention should be pursued for patients with significant functional disability from the disease, >30-degree flexion contracture of the MCP, or any flexion deformity of the PIP. Surgery usually involves fasciectomy. Postponing surgery for too long may result in more permanent loss of extension.

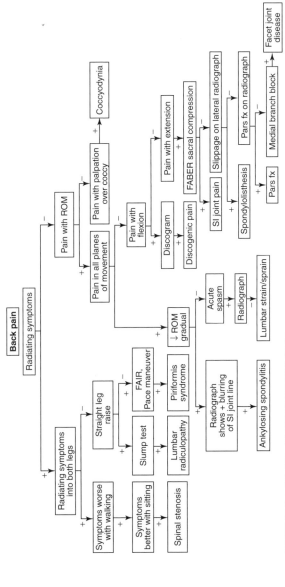

FABER, flexion, abduction, external rotation; FAIR, flexion, adduction, internal rotation; fx, fracture; ROM, range of motion; SI, sacroiliac.

Lower Back and Shooting Leg Pain

5

Red Flag Signs and Symptoms

Any of these signs and symptoms should prompt urgent evaluation and appropriate intervention:

Fevers
Chills
Recent unintended weight loss
Progressive neurologic symptoms
Change in bowel or bladder function
Significant trauma precipitating symptoms

LUMBAR STRAIN/SPRAIN

Background

In much the same way that the mast of a sailboat relies on its supporting standing riggings, the spine relies on all of its supporting muscles and ligaments to maintain its stability. All of these muscles and ligaments can be strained (muscles) and sprained (ligaments). When muscles are imbalanced, weak, or tight, they are more likely to place abnormal biomechanics on the spine and result in acute injury.

Lumbar strain/sprain is probably the most common injury to the lower back. Around 90% of the population at some point in their life has back pain, and >90% of the time the pain resolves on its own without medical intervention. Most of these cases are ascribed to strain/sprain. It is not possible to know if this attribution is accurate. It may be that when a person suffers an acute lower back pain, it is related to the disc. It may be caused by something else such as a sprain/strain. Because it almost always resolves on its own, aggressive diagnosis is not generally indicated in the acute period.

Clinical Presentation

Patients typically recall an inciting event in which they twisted or strained to lift a heavy load that immediately precipitated pain in the lower back. Sometimes, the pain subsides only to worsen at night and then again in the morning. Other times, there is no inciting event and the patient simply wakes up in the morning and describes a pain in the lower back. The pain is usually moderate but may become severe. Most patients wait a few days or more before coming to the doctor. The pain does not radiate and is not associated with any numbness, tingling, or weakness. Sometimes, the pain does refer to the buttocks. When this happens, it refers in a vague, achy pattern. Patients also may report stiffness in the lower back. The pain can be unilateral or bilateral. If the pain has lasted >2 to 3 weeks, it is unlikely to be a simple strain/sprain.

Physical Examination

On examination, the patient may have stiffness in the lower back and be hesitant with movements involving trunk flexion and/or extension. Lumbar lordosis is usually lost because of muscle spasm. Tenderness is typically elicited over the involved area. The muscle is tight, and sometimes a trigger point can be palpated. Trigger points are distinguished from tender points because the former create a referral pain pattern on palpation (tender points are only tender at the exact site of palpation).

Neurologically the patient is intact. Range of motion is intact but hamstrings and hip flexors are often found to be tight.

Diagnostic Studies

Unless any red flags are present, or tenderness is noted over a bony prominence, imaging studies are not routinely ordered in the acute period (within 2 to 3 weeks of onset of symptoms). After 2 to 3 weeks of symptoms, the patient should be investigated for an alternate cause of pain.

Treatment

Reassurance that the pain will most likely go away soon is a large part of initial treatment. Ice and NSAIDs can help in the acute period. In addition, patients should be educated about their backs and how they can take steps to protect their back in the future. An episode of back pain in the past is a predictor of future back pain. Muscle imbalances should be sought and addressed. A brief course of physical therapy is a very good idea for patients. It may speed recovery and it will also teach patients a home exercise program (HEP). The HEP incorporates lumbar stabilization, stretching, and strengthening and is important for the patients to make a part of their daily routine to help them avoid back problems in the future.

Doctors used to recommend absolute bed rest for patients with back pain. Today, this is not the standard of care. Patients should not do activities that exacerbate pain. However, maintaining flexibility and activity is critical to help nourish the structures in the back, speed recovery, and prevent stiffness and further deterioration.

LUMBOSACRAL RADICULITIS/ RADICULOPATHY

Background

Although nowhere near as common as lower back pain, lumbosacral radiculitis is a relatively common problem affecting about 1% of the population. Radiculitis is characterized by inflammation of the nerve root or compression of the dorsal root ganglion. Symptoms include shooting electric pain that *radiates* down from the lower back and/or buttock into the lower extremity. Patients can often take two fingers and trace the distribution of their pain. This is opposed to other referral pain patterns where the pain may be diffuse, vaguely localized, and achy. The symptoms generally follow a characteristic sclerotomal distribution along the nerve root (Fig. 5.1). Lumbosacral radiculopathy is characterized by *loss:* loss of strength, loss of sensation, and/or loss of reflex within the distribution of the involved nerve root(s). Because lumbosacral radiculopathy and radiculitis often coexist and because they are treated the same way, they are often considered as one disorder.

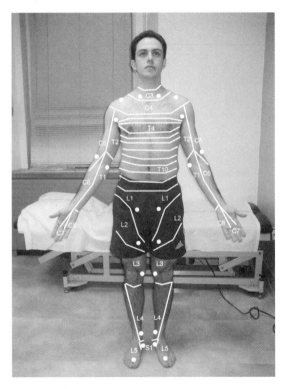

Figure 5.1 Lumbosacral radicular symptoms. Patients can often take two fingers and trace the distribution of their pain. This is opposed to other referral pain patterns where the pain may be diffuse, vaguely localized, and achy. The symptoms generally follow a characteristic sclerotomal distribution along the nerve root.

Note that in the rare instance that neurologic symptoms of a lumbosacral radiculopathy become severe and progressive, or if patients have a sudden change in their bowel or bladder habits (including losing continence), emergent care is necessary and the patient should know to go to the emergency department. Cauda equina syndrome, in which the cauda equina is compressed, may result and is a surgical emergency.

Clinical Presentation

Patients typically present with dull back pain and shooting electric pain that radiates into their lower extremity in a characteristic distribution. Patients sometimes complain of mild weakness (Table 5.1) and/or numbness in their lower extremity. The pain may have come on acutely or developed gradually. Pain may be exacerbated by bending over (in which case a protruded disc is implicated as the cause)

TABLE 5.1
LUMBOSACRAL DISTRIBUTION OF SIGNS AND SYMPTOMS

Root Level	Major Muscle Movements Involved	Reflexes Involved	Deceased Sensation
L2	Hip flexion	None	Medial anterior thigh
L3	Hip flexion, knee extension	Patellar tendon	Medial femoral condyle
L4	Knee extension, ankle dorsiflexion	Patellar tendon	Medial malleolus
L5	Extensor hallucis longus (EHL) extension, hip abduction	Hamstring	EHL
S1	Ankle dorsiflexion and inversion	Achilles	Posterior lateral heel

or with extension (in which case facet hypertrophy is more likely to be the cause). The shooting pains often are intermittent and worse with certain movements.

Physical Examination

Patients may have increased symptoms with lumbar flexion or extension. Straight leg raise (Fig. 5.2) is often positive. In this test the patient lies in the supine position

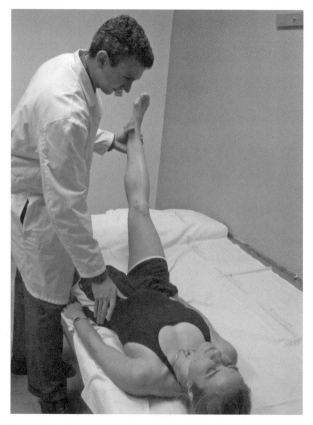

Figure 5.2   Straight leg raise.

and the physician slowly raises the extended leg into the air. Reproduction of radicular symptoms (not hamstring tightness or achy back pain) is a positive test. Passively extending the ankle while the leg is raised may exacerbate symptoms and is highly suggestive of radicular origin.

Seated slump test (Fig. 5.3) is also often positive. In this test, the patient is seated and instructed to drop the chin to the chest and "slump forward." The examiner then passively extends a leg and foot, placing a stress

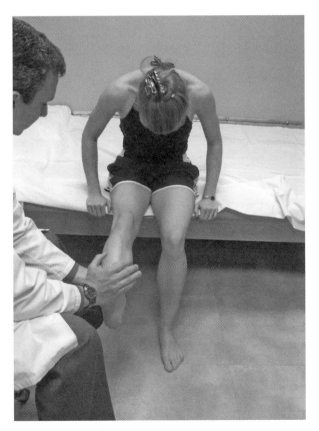

Figure 5.3   Seated slump test.

similar to the straight leg raise. Reproduction of symptoms is a positive test.

Patients may also be found to have numbness and/or weakness along the nerve root(s) that are implicated. Reflexes may be hyporeflexic (Table 5.1).

If an L5 radiculopathy is present, and the patient has a weak gluteus medius, the patient may have a positive Trendelenburg test. In this test, the patient stands on one leg. If the gluteus medius is weak, the patient lurches to that side (Figs. 5.4A and B).

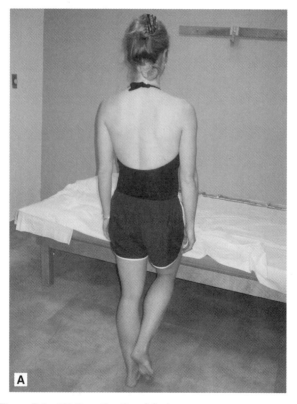

Figure 5.4   (A) Negative Trendelenburg test.

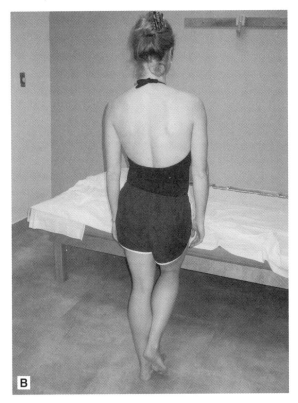

Figure 5.4 (*continued*)   **(B)** Positive Trendelenburg test.

Diagnostic Studies

Radiographs may be obtained and may reveal facet arthropathy, disc space narrowing, or other degenerative changes.

If symptoms are severe, constant, chronic, and/or epidural injections are being considered, magnetic resonance imaging (MRI) should be obtained (Fig. 5.5). The MRI helps delineate the site of nerve root involvement; it helps rule out other pathologies, and it guides injection site.

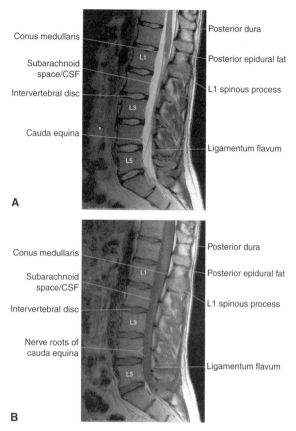

Conus medullaris

Subarachnoid
space/CSF

Intervertebral disc

Cauda equina

Posterior dura

Posterior epidural fat

L1 spinous process

Ligamentum flavum

A

Conus medullaris

Subarachnoid
space/CSF

Intervertebral disc

Nerve roots of
cauda equina

Posterior dura

Posterior epidural fat

L1 spinous process

Ligamentum flavum

B

Figure 5.5 Magnetic resonance imaging—lumbar spine sagittal. (From Berquist T. *MRI of the Musculoskeletal System.* 5th ed. Philadelphia, Pa: Lippincott Williams & Wilkins, 2005, with permission.)

Treatment

The cornerstone of treatment is physical therapy that focuses on lumbar stabilization, increasing hamstring and hip flexor flexibility and strength, and improving postural biomechanics.

Nonsteroidal anti-inflammatory drugs (NSAIDs), analgesics, and muscle relaxants can be helpful depending on the severity of the symptoms. Nerve-stabilizing medications such as gabapentin (e.g., Neurontin) and pregabalin (e.g., Lyrica) can also be helpful to decrease symptoms.

When conservative measures are not sufficient, or if the patient cannot participate in physical therapy because of severe pain, steroids can be used to decrease the inflammation. Some physicians provide an oral steroid taper. These may be effective but are not specifically targeted to the site of inflammation and have greater systemic side effects.

A fluoroscopically guided epidural steroid injection can be very effective. The injection can be performed via either a transforaminal, interlaminar, or caudal route depending on the nerve roots involved. For most instances, the transforaminal route is favored.

If MRI reveals a contained disc bulge or protrusion to be causing symptoms, and if epidural steroid injection(s) and physical therapy do not treat the symptoms adequately, a percutaneous microdiscectomy or nucleoplasty may be appropriate. This procedure serves to essentially debulk or "shrink" the disc, thus taking the pressure off of the nerve root.

Persistent, debilitating symptoms despite aggressive nonsurgical care should prompt a surgical evaluation. Surgical options include discectomy and discectomy with fusion.

If the patient has progressive neurologic symptoms and/or bowel or bladder changes, a high index of suspicion must be maintained for cauda equina syndrome, which is a surgical emergency.

DISCOGENIC LOWER BACK PAIN

Background

Perhaps no other common diagnosis causes as much controversy or strife as the discogenic lower back. This need not be the case. The confusion stems from equating discogenic lower back pain with a herniated disc. As in the cervical and thoracic spine, the disc can be likened to a jelly donut. There is an inner jelly (nucleus pulposus) and an outer crust (annulus fibrosus). There are no nerve fibers in the nucleus pulposus. The nerve fibers, which are capable of transmitting painful signals, are located in the outer third (and occasionally two-thirds) of the annulus fibrosus. When these nerves are irritated either from mechanical or chemical irritation, the disc is the source of back pain.

For the annular nerve fibers to be irritated, a tear must exist in the annulus fibrosus that extends to the nucleus pulposus. This tear allows the inflammatory mediators such as tumor necrosis factor alpha and interleukins, which are within the nucleus pulposus, to seep out and irritate the annular nerve fibers. Then, when the disc is loaded with pressure, these irritated nerve fibers that are bathed in chemical inflammatory mediators are likely to cause pain.

Discogenic lower back pain is the number-one cause of chronic (lasting >3 months) back pain. It may be relatively more common in younger people (accounting for roughly 40%), but it is still an important cause in older people (30% to 40% of cases).

Clinical Presentation

Patients may recall an acute injury such as opening a window, leg-pressing a heavy weight, or bending to pick up a paper that precipitated the pain. The inciting event usually involves trunk flexion. Sometimes, the pain occurs more gradually and no inciting event is noted.

Patients typically present with axial lower back pain that may refer into the buttocks or as far down as the knee. The pain is typically worse with prolonged sitting and with bending over. This is because flexion increases the load on the disc. Patients often report increased pain in the morning (studies indicate that because of gravity and hormonal factors, there is increased pressure in the discs in the morning). The character of pain is often dull and achy, although it may be sharp. Shooting leg pain, numbness, and weakness are *not* characteristic.

Physical Examination

Pain may be exacerbated with trunk flexion and patients may be hesitant to bend over for this reason. The patient is neurologically intact. Hamstrings and hip flexors are often found to be tight. Otherwise, the examination is often unremarkable.

Diagnostic Studies

Radiographs may be obtained and may reveal degenerative changes in the spine as well as more pronounced decreased disc height at the level involved. An MRI is the most useful imaging test. The decision to obtain one is based on how aggressive the physician and patient want to be with treatment. MRI may reveal decreased disc height at the level involved. MRI T2 images (which light up more for inflammation) may also reveal a high-intensity zone (HIZ) in the annulus of the disc. However, annular HIZ zones are not diagnostic. In fact, it is important to note that no imaging study is capable of diagnosing discogenic back pain. The gold standard for diagnosing lumbar discogenic disease is lumbar discography.

Treatment

The cornerstone of treatment for degenerative disc disease, as with most causes of lower back pain, is physical therapy to focus on core strengthening, lumbar stabilization, stretching of hamstrings and hip flexors, and correcting any muscle imbalances. For discogenic pain, the therapy should have an extension bias. NSAIDs may also be helpful. Ice can also be used to help reduce inflammation.

Wearing a back brace or lumbar support during heavy lifting may be appropriate. However, a lumbar support does not provide lumbar stability but only serves as a reminder for patients to maintain proper posture and precautions.

When physical therapy and medications are not effective in alleviating symptoms, more invasive treatment may be needed. Fluoroscopically guided epidural steroid injections may be performed. If the epidural steroid injection(s) is not effective, intradiscal electrothermal therapy (IDET) is another alternative in younger patients with well-maintained disc heights. IDET involves placing a catheter into the annulus of the disc over the tear under fluoroscopic guidance. The catheter is then heated causing collagen and nerve denaturing. Patients are placed in a molded brace after the procedure for about 6 to 8 weeks. It may take this amount of time for the patient to experience pain relief. It is important to tell patients that their pain may actually increase in the first few days or even weeks following the procedure. However, in appropriately selected patients (preserved disc height, no instability, contained disc), the procedure may have a 75% efficacy rate.

When aggressive conservative care does not sufficiently alleviate symptoms, surgical options may be considered. The two main surgical procedures include artificial disc replacement and fusion surgery. Many patients may obtain relief from both surgical interventions, however, and the belief is that an artificial disc may maintain physiologic movement and loading in the spine better than a fusion. An added benefit of disc replacement is that if it fails, fusion surgery can still be performed.

FACET JOINT SYNDROME (Z-JOINT DISEASE)

Background

Lumbar facets are the second most common cause of chronic lower back pain. They account for approximately 40% of cases in older patients and 15% to 20% in younger patients. Facet joints are synovial joints in the spine that facilitate flexion and extension and resist forward sliding and twisting. Like other synovial joints, they can become injured, arthritic, and painful.

Clinical Presentation

Patients are typically older than 50 years (although they can be any age) and present with axial back pain that may refer as low as the buttock or even knee. Rarely, the pain may refer to the lower leg and foot. Referral pain patterns are a deep, aching pain that is vague in distribution. Pain is typically worse with standing for prolonged periods of time and walking and climbing down stairs (although not necessarily up stairs). Pain is better with sitting and bending forward. The patient does not typically recall an inciting event, but rather the pain tends to come on gradually.

Physical Examination

Patients characteristically have pain with trunk extension. Oblique extension may be more painful in the direction of the patient's pain (Fig. 5.6). The rest of the examination is likely to be unremarkable. The overlying back muscles may be tender and/or stiff.

Diagnostic Studies

Radiographs may be obtained and may reveal arthritic changes in the facet joints. MRI likewise may show arthritic changes and possibly inflammation within the facets. However, importantly, radiograph, computed tomography (CT), and MRI have not been shown to diagnose facet joint pain reliably. Recently, bone scan with single-photon emission computed tomography (SPECT) has proven to be promising for diagnosing facet mediated pain. This approach is still being developed, and further studies are needed.

Fluoroscopic-guided medial branch blocks remain the gold-standard diagnostic approach to diagnose facet joint syndrome reliably. When single blocks are performed, there may be a 25% false-positive rate. This rate drops to <15% when double-blind blocks are used. In double-blind blocks, the facet joint is injected once with a short-acting anesthetic (e.g., lidocaine) and at a different time with a longer acting anesthetic (e.g., bupivacaine).

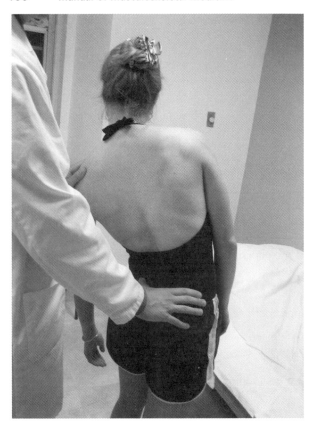

Figure 5.6 Lumbar trunk oblique extension.

Treatment

When patients are identified with suspected facet joint pain, physical therapy focusing on core stabilization and medications are the usual first step. If this fails, an intra-articular injection of anesthetic and corticosteroid is appropriate. It is often difficult to determine *which* facet is implicated, and multiple facets may need to be injected. This injection can be used for diagnostic as well as therapeutic reasons. If the patient receives relief from the injection, the facets can reasonably be believed to be the pain generator.

Once the diagnosis has been confirmed, if the steroid injection does not provide lasting relief, it can be repeated, or radiofrequency neurotomy of the medial branches supplying the facet joints can be performed. If a repeat injection also does not provide lasting relief, radiofrequency neurotomy should be pursued.

Radiofrequency neurotomy is a percutaneous procedure performed under fluoroscopic guidance. In it, radiofrequency energy is used essentially to heat and ablate the nerves supplying the facets.

SACROILIAC JOINT PAIN

Background

The sacroiliac (SI) joint is the cause of chronic lower back pain in about 10% to 15% of cases. Ventral capsular tears in the tough joint capsule may contribute to the pathologic mechanism, but the exact pathophysiology is not known. Some physicians, chiropractors, and therapists may report hypermobility as the source of SI pain. This may be the case; however, biomechanical and radiographic data have shown that even SI joints diagnosed with hypermobility have relatively little movement. Micromotion leading to malalignment and joint inflammation is believed to be a part of the pain complex. If there are differences in mobility that are affecting pain, they are very subtle and difficult to detect. SI joint pain remains a controversial diagnosis in certain circles, with some believing it represents a higher percentage of pain and some believing it represents less than the documented 10% to 15%.

Clinical Presentation

Patients typically present with pain on or around the SI joint. The pain can be unilateral or bilateral. Sometimes the pain refers to the buttocks and thighs. Occasionally the pain radiates up into the middle back. The pain is usually dull and achy, although sometimes the pain can be described as sharp. Pregnant women are more likely to experience this condition because of the laxity of ligaments during pregnancy caused by hormonal factors.

Physical Examination

Maneuvers that stress the SI joint are not diagnostic of themselves, but they form part of the picture of SI joint pain. Interestingly, when a patient points to the SI joint when asked where the pain is located, this is a sensitive indicator that the patient's source of pain is the SI joint.

Hip end-range internal and external rotation may cause pain in the SI joint. The FABER (*f*lexion, *ab*duction, *ex*ternal *r*otation) test (also called the Patrick test) (Fig. 5.7) is often positive. In this test, the patient lies supine and the knee is flexed to 90 degrees and the hip externally rotated so the ankle of that leg rests on the contralateral knee. The physician then applies a force pushing down on the flexed knee and contralateral anterior superior iliac spine. Reproduction of symptoms with this maneuver implicates the SI joint as the pain generator.

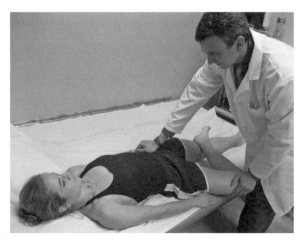

Figure 5.7 FABER (Patrick) test.

The SI compression test is another good examination maneuver. In this test, the patient lies prone and the physician applies a downward force onto the SI joint. Reproduction of symptoms is considered a positive test.

Diagnostic Studies

Radiographs may be obtained and may reveal arthritic changes in the SI joint. MRI may also be obtained. Neither radiographs or MRI are diagnostic of SI joint pain. However, they are often obtained to exclude other causes and also because many physicians feel they are necessary before performing intra-articular injections, which is the gold-standard diagnostic test.

Under fluoroscopic guidance, an intra-articular injection anesthetic is placed into the SI joint. When this relieves the pain, it is considered diagnostic. Corticosteroid is often added to the injectate to offer a therapeutic potential.

Treatment

Physical therapy is the cornerstone of therapy. Lumbar stabilization, correcting muscle imbalances, stretching, and strengthening are all part of the therapy prescription. Ice can also be useful to reduce inflammation. An SI joint belt can be worn and is sometimes effective. Some physicians believe SI joint periligamentous injections with lidocaine and/or corticosteroids are helpful. Osteopathic manipulations have also been reported by some physicians to be helpful.

When more conservative measures are not effective, a fluoroscopically guided injection of steroid and anesthetic into the joint space can be performed. This is often done as part of establishing the diagnosis.

Surgical options are limited. In the past, the SI joint has been fused. This is not a good treatment for most patients because the fused joint often leads to an adjacent stress fracture or, also commonly, other parts of the spine become painful with the abnormal biomechanics placed on the spine by SI fusion.

SI joint pain in pregnant women and postpartum women who are nursing should be managed very conservatively. The pain typically resolves after pregnancy. Injections should not be performed. Gentle osteopathic manipulations by an experienced expert physician may be helpful in peripartum and postpartum patients who are nursing but still have pain.

SPINAL STENOSIS

Background

Spinal stenosis refers to the narrowing of the central spinal bony canal that houses the spinal cord and nerve roots. Narrowing of the canal usually occurs because of the degenerative changes that occur in the spine, which include facet hypertrophy, disc bulges, protrusions, and ligament hypertrophy. Stenosis can also be caused by slippage of one vertebral body on another. All of these changes that occur to the spine result in the narrowing of the bony canal, which ultimately results in nerve or spinal cord compression.

Clinical Presentation

Patients with spinal stenosis usually complain of a gradual onset of pain that worsens with standing and/or walking. A good gauge of the severity of spinal stenosis is the distance a patient can tolerate walking. Patients also report much relief with sitting as opposed to standing. They often compensate and walk in a stooped position to achieve some pain relief while walking. Pain is usually bilateral and accompanied by numbness and tingling.

Physical Examination

On physical examination patients usual present walking in a stooped position. Range of motion testing usually worsens pain with extension. All other provocative maneuvers, such as straight leg raising, are usually negative. Neurologic testing reveals some sensory deficits and difficulty with tandem ambulation in advanced cases.

Diagnostic Studies

The gold standard for detecting spinal stenosis is an MRI. Radiographs and CT scan also give some information regarding the bony structures.

Treatment

The first step in treating spinal stenosis involves medications and physical therapy. A course of NSAIDs, nerve stabilizers such as Neurontin and Lyrica, and opioids may be used depending on the severity of the pain. If patients continue to experience continued debilitating pain, a series of epidural injections should be considered.

Once all conservative treatment options are exhausted, surgical intervention should be pursued. If the spine is stable a laminectomy may be sufficient in treating the pain. If there is instability noted, laminectomy with fusion is the better option.

ANKYLOSING SPONDYLITIS

Background

Ankylosing spondylitis (AS) is a spondyloarthropathy that primarily affects the spine and sacroiliac joints. The eyes (iritis, uveitis), heart (aortitis), feet (plantar fasciitis), lungs (pulmonary fibrosis), and bowels (inflammatory bowel disease) can all be affected, as can other parts of the body. Patients with AS need at least annual checkups with an ophthalmologist, and should have their overall care directed by a physician familiar with the disease. There is a male predilection for the disease (3:1), and peak onset is between 15 and 35 years of age.

Clinical Presentation

The classic presentation is a young man (20 to 30 years of age) who presents with gradual onset back pain that is worse in the morning and gets better as the day goes on. Activity makes the pain *better* and rest makes it *worse*. The pain is typically located over the sacroiliac joints. Rib cage pain may also be present when taking a deep breath or coughing.

Physical Examination

Physical examination should be consistent with sacroiliac joint pain (see section on SI joint pain). In addition, range of motion may be restricted throughout the spine.

Diagnostic Studies

Patients are sometimes investigated for the antigen HLA-B27. Approximately 90% of patients with AS have this antigen; however, it is very nonspecific for the disease (approximately 5% of the population have the antigen but not the disease). People with HLA-B27 have about a 1% to 2% risk of developing the disease, compared with 0.1% to 0.2% in the general population in the United States. HLA-B27 may also correlate with other pathologies such as reactive arthritis and psoriatic arthritis.

The diagnostic hallmark of the disease is inflammation (blurring of the joint line) and/or fusion of the sacroiliac joints seen on radiograph. Squaring of the vertebral bodies may also be seen.

CT and MRI also may be helpful as part of the workup for the disease and for evaluating associated fractures and other pathologies, but history, physical examination, and radiographs are usually enough to make the diagnosis.

Treatment

Early diagnosis and education about the condition are an important part of treatment. NSAIDs can be useful for pain and inflammation. Because back pain is often the initial presenting symptom of AS, the musculoskeletal or family practice physician is often the first to see the patient. The patient will require referral to a physician used to managing a patient with AS to ensure proper monitoring of potential heart, lung, neurologic, and eye problems.

Fluoroscopic sacroiliac joint injections of steroid and anesthetic may be helpful for the acute back pain. All patients should also undergo a course of physical therapy. Incorporating a stretching and strengthening program into the patient's daily routine will be important in preventing long-term problems and disability.

PARS INTERARTICULARIS FRACTURE (LUMBAR SPONDYLOLYSIS)

Background

A relatively common cause of lower back pain in the younger athlete is a pars interarticularis stress fracture, most typically at the L5-S1 level. These fractures can be unilateral or bilateral. When bilateral, they may result in spondylolisthesis. Although more common in younger athletes, they can occur and cause pain at any age. The presence of a pars interarticularis stress fracture must be correlated with symptoms because many or most of these stress fractures may be asymptomatic.

Clinical Presentation

Patients typically present with lower back pain that is unilateral or bilateral. The pain may be sharp or dull. The pain may have begun acutely after a fall or sudden movement, or it may have developed slowly over time. Patients typically report a history of repetitive extension activities such as participation in gymnastics, swimming, dancing, or football. As the pain increases, the patient may report that he or she can no longer participate in their sport.

Physical Examination

The classic finding is a positive stork test. In this test, the patient stands on the foot of the most painful side and obliquely extends the trunk over the painful side. When this reproduces symptoms, it is considered positive.

Tenderness to palpation over the involved region may also be present. If spondylolisthesis is present, a step-off may be present on palpation of the spinous processes.

Diagnostic Studies

Lumbar radiographs should be obtained. The pars interarticularis is best viewed as the neck or collar of the "Scotty dog" on the oblique film. If positive, the "Scotty dog" has a broken neck (Fig. 5.8). Of note, oblique radiographs require considerably more radiation exposure than do anteroposterior and lateral films. Therefore, they should only be ordered when necessary.

If the lumbar radiographs are normal but clinical suspicion remains high, bone scan with SPECT may be a superior method for evaluating the potential lesion.

Treatment

The cornerstone of treatment in the acutely painful period of a pars interarticularis fracture is bracing, icing, and physical therapy to work on strengthening as well as stretching the hip flexors and extensors. The brace, typically a Boston overlapping brace, lumbar corset, or Warm-n-Form orthosis, prevents hyperextension and is worn for 23 hours per day until the patient remains asymptomatic for 3 months. After this time, repeat imaging is obtained to demonstrate healing. Unfortunately, patient compliance for wearing the brace is low.

Patients with persistent pain despite bracing and therapy may benefit from a fluoroscopically guided block of the medial branch supplying the painful area to confirm the diagnosis. Once confirmed as the pain generator, a

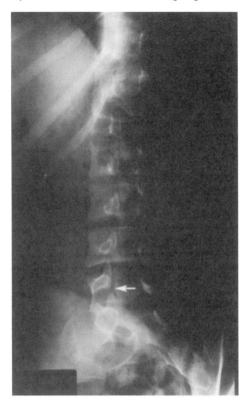

Figure 5.8   Radiograph of Scotty dog with broken neck. (From Birrer R, Griesmer B, Cataletto M. *Pediatric Sports Medicine for Primary Care*. Philadelphia, Pa: Lippincott Williams & Wilkins, 2002, with permission.)

radiofrequency rhizotomy can be performed to sever the nerve supply to the painful area. Long-term follow-up data for this procedure for this diagnosis are not available, and so it should be done only when absolutely necessary and the patient does not respond to more conservative measures. Surgery is rarely necessary, but surgical options are also available and include direct repair of the fracture, repair and fusion of the segment, and removal of the segment.

SPONDYLOLISTHESIS

Background

Spondylolisthesis is generally an asymptomatic finding on radiograph, but it can also cause symptoms in some patients. Spondylolisthesis refers to a slippage of one vertebral body in relation to an adjacent one. It is graded in terms of severity: grade I, 1% to 25% slippage; grade II, 26% to 50%; grade III, 51% to 75%; and grade IV, >75% slippage. The most common cause of spondylolisthesis in the young athlete is a pars interarticularis fracture at the L5-S1 level. In older patients, degenerative changes to the disc and facet joints are the most common cause for spondylolisthesis.

Clinical Presentation

When spondylolisthesis is symptomatic, patients generally report lower back pain that is exacerbated by lumbar extension. Occasionally, patients may report radicular symptoms if a nerve root is impinged and inflamed. (See section on lumbosacral radiculitis for details on this pathology).

Physical Examination

If the spondylolisthesis is large enough, a step-off may be noted on palpation of the spinous processes. Hamstring tightness is often noted. Pain may be exacerbated with trunk extension and trunk oblique extension. A thorough neurologic evaluation should be performed to help rule out lumbosacral radicular involvement.

Diagnostic Studies

Radiographs are typically sufficient to evaluate spondylolisthesis. Flexion and extension views should be obtained to assess for instability.

Bone scan with SPECT and/or CT scan also may be obtained, particularly if evaluating for a spondylolysis.

Treatment

Asymptomatic grade I slips require no treatment. They should be followed with routine radiographs until growth is completed to monitor the slip. Asymptomatic grade II and III slips require no treatment, but patients should be advised against repetitive extension activities (e.g., gymnastics), occupations that require heavy manual labor, and contact sports.

Symptomatic grades I and II slips can be treated conservatively with alteration of activities to avoid repetitive hyperextension and contact sports, participation in physical therapy to focus on core stabilization in a flexion based program, as well as exercises to increase hamstring flexibility. Symptomatic grade III and IV slips should be evaluated by a surgeon for possible surgical intervention. Symptomatic grade I and II slips that do not respond to aggressive conservative care may also be surgical candidates, although this is rarely necessary.

PIRIFORMIS SYNDROME

Background

The sciatic nerve passes either inferior, around, or through the piriformis muscle. When the sciatic nerve is irritated by the piriformis muscle, it is termed *piriformis syndrome.* Piriformis syndrome remains a controversial diagnosis with some physicians believing it is underdiagnosed and others equally convinced it is overdiagnosed. Many physicians believe it accounts for 5% to 10% of all cases of "sciatica" (patients complaining of shooting leg pain).

Clinical Presentation

Patients typically present with buttock pain and shooting pain that radiates in an S1 distribution down the back of the thigh and leg. Sometimes, it also may radiate in an L5 distribution down the lateral thigh into the lateral lower leg. The radiating pain is often characterized as "burning," "shooting," and/or "electric." Patients also sometimes complain of lower back pain. Patients also may have numbness in the distribution of symptoms. Symptoms are often exacerbated by walking or sitting.

Physical Examination

The hallmark physical examination finding is marked tenderness over the piriformis in the buttock as the sciatic nerve crosses near (or through) it. When palpation at this point also reproduces the patient's symptoms radiating into the lower extremity, it is very suggestive of piriformis syndrome.

Symptoms also may be reproduced with FAIR (*f*lexion, *a*dduction, *i*nternal *r*otation) while the patient is in the contralateral decubitus position (Fig. 5.9). The Pace maneuver is another test that is useful for diagnosing piriformis syndrome. With the affected leg in the FAIR position, the patient is instructed to abduct the hip against resistance. This maneuver causes the piriformis muscle to contract. An increase in pain with resisted abduction is considered a positive test.

Weakness is not typically encountered, but when present it will be in an L5 and/or S1 distribution. Resisted external rotation and abduction of the hip may reveal weakness, although this "weakness" must be differentiated from pain causing weakness. When this resistance reproduces symptoms, it is called a positive Pace sign.

Diagnostic Studies

Radiographs are sometimes obtained but do not yield diagnostic information in piriformis syndrome.

MRI of the lumbosacral spine is helpful to obtain to help rule out a radicular cause of symptoms. Also, MRI of the pelvis can be obtained if a mass is suspected of compressing the sciatic nerve.

Electromyelography/nerve conduction velocity studies can be helpful to differentiate the site of nerve compression, if present.

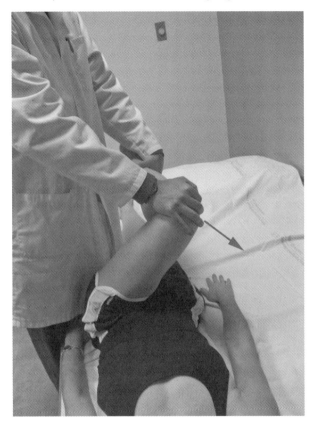

Figure 5.9   FAIR test.

Treatment

Physical therapy is the cornerstone of treatment. Therapy should emphasize stretching of the piriformis muscle. Modalities prior to stretching may be helpful. Soft tissue mobilization techniques are also helpful. Core stabilization exercises should also be performed.

Trigger point injection using corticosteroid and anesthetic as part of the injection performed over the point of maximal tenderness in the buttock (assuming this point was found on physical examination) is often helpful. Dry needling also can be used.

Some physicians also inject botulinum toxin A (e.g., Botox) into the muscle to treat piriformis spasm.

Surgical release of the piriformis is rarely indicated but can be effective in patients resistant to aggressive conservative care.

COCCYDYNIA

Background

Coccydynia refers to pain over the coccyx. It is more common in women than men. Common etiologies include postpartum and trauma to the coccyx (often from a fall). About a third of coccydynia cases are believed to be idiopathic.

Clinical Presentation

Patients complain of pain over their coccyx. The pain often begins immediately after a trauma such as a fall or having been kicked in the coccyx. The pain also may begin after childbirth. It can also occur as a result of prolonged sitting or simply begin gradually without any inciting event. Sitting is painful in patients with coccydynia.

Physical Examination

The hallmark physical examination finding is reproduction of symptoms with palpation of the coccyx and/or the sacrococcygeal joint. A step-off may also be noted while palpating the coccyx indicating possible dislocation of the coccyx.

Diagnostic Studies

Radiographs may be obtained to rule out a coccygeal dislocation or fracture. With dislocation the coccyx may be seen forming a 90-degree angle in relation to the sacrum. Standing and sitting studies may be obtained to assess coccygeal mobility.

Treatment

Conservative care includes using a donut-shaped pillow or gel cushion to relieve the pressure on the coccyx.

Manipulation of the coccyx and trying to relax the surrounding soft tissues manually have been performed with limited success.

A steroid and anesthetic injection into the coccyx is often very effective. Optimally, the injection is performed under ultrasound or fluoroscopic guidance.

Recently, the ganglion impar, which is part of the sympathetic nervous system and located directly anterior to the sacral-coccygeal junction, has been injected under fluoroscopic guidance with promising results. More research is needed to identify the true efficacy of this treatment.

Surgery is rarely necessary. However, when aggressive conservative care is not successful, surgical options include performing a limited coccygectomy, which can be very effective when patients are properly selected.

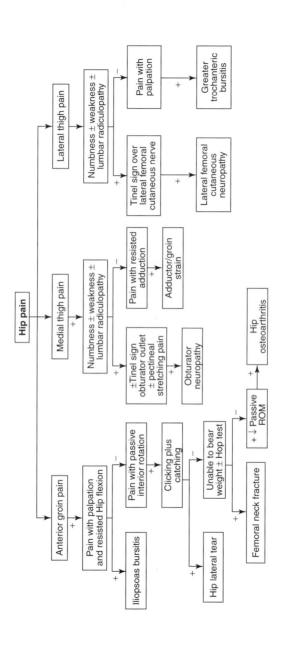

Hip and Groin Pain

6

> **Red Flag Signs and Symptoms**
>
> Any of these signs and symptoms should prompt urgent evaluation and appropriate intervention:
>
> Fevers
> Chills
> Hot, swollen joint
> Progressive neurologic symptoms
> Loss of pulses

GROIN STRAIN

Background

The muscles of the inner thigh consist of the adductor magnus, adductor longus, and adductor brevis. This muscle group is commonly injured in sports that require lateral movement or pivoting. Sudden forced abduction of the hip usually causes injury to the inner thigh or groin. Usually minor tears occur in the muscle belly causing severe pain.

Clinical Presentation

Usually patients present with pain localized to the inner thigh. Depending on the severity of the injury, patients may complain of difficulty with sport-specific activity, normal walking, or at rest. Pain is exacerbated by lateral movement or pivoting.

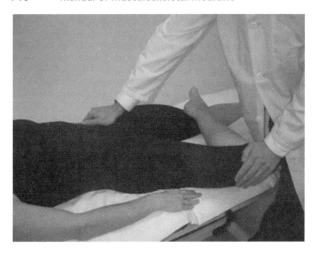

Figure 6.1   FABER (Patrick) test.

Physical Examination

The patient's pain is usually elicited with resisted adduction. The FABER (*f*lexion *ab*duction *e*xternal *r*otation) (Patrick) test (Fig. 6.1) also reproduces the patient's pain. In addition, palpation of the muscle may reproduce the patient's pain. Examination of ambulation may reveal an antalgic gait.

Diagnostic Studies

Usually imaging studies are not needed to diagnose strain. If the pain persists after an adequate amount of rest, physical therapy, ice, and medication, magnetic resonance imaging (MRI) may be needed to assess the soft tissue.

Treatment

Rest, ice, compression, and elevation (RICE) is the initial treatment of any strain. Usually patients are instructed to rest for 4 to 6 weeks to allow moderate to severe strains to heal. Medications such as anti-inflammatories are useful in treating pain and the inflammation that may be present. If the pain continues despite adequate rest, the use of a thigh sleeve to help contain the muscle is effective.

HIP OSTEOARTHRITIS

Background

As many as 25% of people may develop hip osteoarthritis (OA) at some point in their life according to the Johnston County Osteoarthritis Project. This risk is increased in people who are overweight or obese. Previous trauma to the hip also increases risk. As in other body parts, osteoarthritis is characterized by articular cartilage loss.

Clinical Presentation

Patients classically present with groin pain. The pain also may refer into the anterior thigh, buttock, or knee. Pain is initially aggravated by walking and climbing stairs. As the disease progresses, pain may be present at rest and nighttime. Patients may complain of limping because of the pain.

Physical Examination

An antalgic gait may be noted with the patient favoring the uninvolved side. The hallmark physical examination finding is loss of internal rotation as well as reproduction of symptoms with internal rotation and external rotation. Range of motion while loading the joint is also a good test. For this examination maneuver, the patient lies supine and the physician rotates the hip internally and externally while compressing the femur into the acetabulum with a downward pressure on the knee.

Diagnostic Studies

Radiographs should be obtained and may reveal asymmetric joint space narrowing, osteophytes, subchondral cyst, and/or sclerosis (Fig. 6.2). Importantly, radiographic findings do not necessarily correlate with severity of disease. Radiographs may reveal significant arthritis but the patient may have minimal symptoms. Reciprocally, radiographs may be normal and symptoms significant.

MRI may be more sensitive and specific for osteoarthritis in terms of evaluating the cartilage. However, this costly test is not practical or needed in most cases of hip OA.

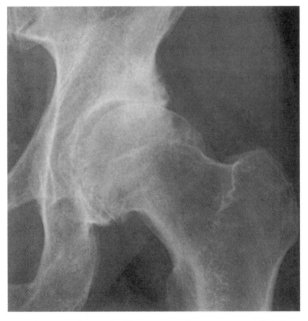

Figure 6.2   Radiograph of hip osteoarthritis. (From Moskowitz et al. *Osteoarthritis Diagnosis and Medical/Surgical Management.* 4th ed. Philadelphia, Pa: Lippincott Williams & Wilkins, 2007, with permission.)

Treatment

Physical therapy is the cornerstone of treatment. When a hip becomes arthritic and painful, the patient's inclination may be not to use it. However, disuse does not allow needed nourishment to get to the remaining cartilage, leading to further quickening cartilage loss. Physical therapy works on strengthening the supporting musculature of the hip, as well as improving core stabilization, and addresses any flexibility limitations.

The patient should be encouraged to listen to their body but try and stay active. Weightbearing exercises that are nonimpact are ideal. Using an elliptical machine is an excellent example. Alternatively, nonweightbearing exercises are also good. These would include swimming or riding the stationery bike. Impact exercises are all right to do and are certainly better than doing no exercises, but they may be too painful. Patients must listen to their body to help guide them in terms of which exercises to perform.

Nonsteroidal anti-inflammatory drugs (NSAIDs) and acetaminophen can also be helpful for mild pain relief. Oral supplementation with glucosamine and chondroitin sulfate and topical analgesic creams may also be helpful.

Intra-articular injections of corticosteroid and anesthetic can be very effective in reducing symptoms of hip OA. The injections should be done under fluoroscopic or ultrasound guidance. Ideally, the injection (as well as all analgesic medications) is used as a bridge to reduce the pain and allow the patient to participate more fully with physical therapy. Intra-articular hyaluronic acid injections also appear promising in treating hip OA, although more research is needed.

When symptoms become progressive and not responsive to aggressive conservative care, surgical options are available. Although hip fusion is one option, total hip replacement is the preferred surgical procedure. Total hip replacement makes dramatic improvements in quality of life for patients who need it. Total hip replacements can be done using cement or cementless techniques. Hybrid procedures using both cementless and cemented parts are also available. In general, younger patients with healthy bones are offered the cementless replacements. Older patients, or patients with weak bones or rheumatoid arthritis, are typically offered the cemented replacements. Of course, patients should have a full discussion of all the risks and benefits of the different prosthesis options with their surgeon.

HIP LABRAL TEAR

Background

The labrum is a fibrocartilaginous ring structure that encompasses and deepens the acetabulum of the hip. It functions as an interface and cushioning structure between the femoral head and the acetabulum. Like other fibrocartilaginous structures, the labrum of the hip is subject to injury, which usually occurs from repetitive stress from high-impact activities. This injury is usually seen in runners and dancers.

Clinical Presentation

Patients typically present with complaints similar to hip OA. The primary differences are that patients with a hip labral tear are more likely to be younger and have episodes of hip clicking, popping, or possibly feeling that the hip is "going to give out." However, as with hip OA, the typical complaints include groin pain. Patients may also have anterior thigh pain. Walking and other weightbearing activities tend to exacerbate the symptoms. The pain may or may not have been precipitated by a traumatic insult such as having suffered a fall, twisting, or pivot injury.

Physical Examination

On examination, patients may or may not have pain with internal and external range of motion of the hip. The more characteristic physical examination finding is for patients to have pain with hip flexion and adduction. When hip

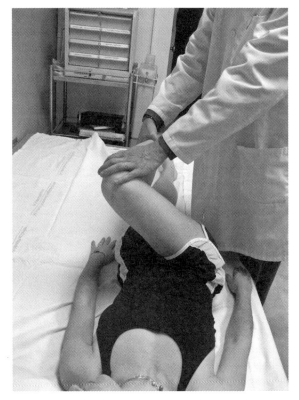

Figure 6.3 Hip flexion and adduction.

flexion and adduction (Fig. 6.3) reproduce groin symptoms but internal and external range of motion manipulation does not, the patient is likely to have a labral tear.

Diagnostic Studies

Radiographs are important to obtain. They may show an absence of arthritic changes, which does not rule out hip OA but does suggest another etiology may be present. MRI alone is not very sensitive (about 80%) or specific (about 65%) for labral tears. MRI with arthrogram has a <90% sensitivity and specificity for hip labral tears.

If the diagnosis remains in doubt, an intra-articular hip injection of anesthetic medication can be performed under ultrasound or fluoroscopic guidance. If this injection removes the symptoms temporarily, the pathology is intra-articular. Steroid is often added to the injectate to offer a potential therapeutic effect.

The gold-standard diagnostic procedure to diagnose hip labral tears remains hip arthroscopy.

Treatment

Importantly, acetabular labral tears may occur in asymptomatic patients. Treatment is only necessary if symptoms are present.

Conservative care for acetabular labral tears includes physical therapy that focuses on stretching and strengthening the surrounding hip musculature. Core stabilization is also helpful. NSAIDs may also be useful.

Intra-articular steroid and anesthetic injection performed under fluoroscopic or ultrasound guidance may also be helpful. This should be done in conjunction with physical therapy.

Hip arthroscopy is a good surgical alternative for large symptomatic acetabular labral tears. In addition, a bucket-handle tear may not respond as well to more conservative measures.

LATERAL FEMORAL CUTANEOUS NERVE ENTRAPMENT (MERALGIA PARESTHETICA)

Background

The lateral femoral cutaneous nerve is, suggested by its name, a purely sensory nerve. It is actually not a branch of the femoral nerve but rather arises from the posterior branches of L2 and L3. The nerve supplies the skin of the anterior-lateral thigh.

Clinical Presentation

Patients typically present with paresthesias, including numbness, tingling, and/or burning running down the anterior-lateral aspect of the thigh from just medial and inferior to the anterior superior iliac spine (ASIS) laterally to above the lateral knee. Patients may also have hypoesthesia in this region. Symptoms may be exacerbated with hip extension, and patients may note this while jogging or using an elliptical machine in the gym.

Patients may report a recent increase of abdominal girth (a tight belt can cause this entrapment) or pregnancy. Other patients may report wearing a tight tool belt daily at work. Still others simply note that the symptoms started without any inciting event, including no increased weight or tight belts. It is also seen in diabetics.

Physical Examination

The classic examination finding is reproduction of symptoms with palpation directly medial to, or inferior to, the ASIS while the hip is held in extension. Decreased sensation may also be noted over the distribution of the nerve. A full neurologic examination must be performed because one of the principal differential diagnoses is a lumbosacral radiculitis.

Diagnostic Studies

In uncomplicated cases, this is primarily a clinical diagnosis.

Imaging studies are not helpful to diagnose this entrapment directly (they may be helpful to rule out others). Side-to-side comparison of the nerve conduction study of the lateral femoral cutaneous nerve is a useful diagnostic tool. Electromyelography/nerve conduction velocity (EMG/NCV) studies may also be helpful to rule out other causes such as radiculopathy or plexopathy.

A local anesthetic injection immediately inferior to the ASIS over the nerve may eliminate symptoms and confirm the diagnosis.

Treatment

Initial treatment includes education about the entrapment and physical therapy. If a tight belt is implicated as the cause, wearing a looser belt may be sufficient to take away the symptoms. Of course, the patient should also be advised to lose weight if appropriate. During therapy, modalities may be helpful for this condition, including a transcutaneous electrical nerve stimulator, ultrasound, moist heat, and soft tissue massage. However, the cornerstone of therapy remains stretching and strengthening the surrounding musculature.

A steroid and anesthetic injection over the nerve near the ASIS may be helpful to relieve more chronic symptoms.

Rarely, surgical decompression of the nerve may be necessary.

OBTURATOR NEUROPATHY

Background

The obturator nerve arises from the second, third, and fourth lumbar nerve roots. It then travels through the psoas muscle and emerges through the obturator canal to innervate the adductor muscles. Injury to this nerve usually occurs due to twisting, kicking, and running. The exact mechanism of injury is not clear, but it is believed the injury occurs at the outlet of the obturator foramen.

Clinical Presentation

Patients usually complain of pain with some associated numbness in the medial thigh. Pain is localized to the groin or inner thigh region. Exacerbating factors include walking, kicking, or pivoting. The pain is sometimes described as burning or sharp. Patients may have difficulties with ambulation.

Physical Examination

Pain is usually elicited with resisted hip flexion or adduction. Weakness may also be seen depending on the severity of the syndrome. Paresthesias or numbness in the distribution of the obturator nerve may be seen. The Patrick test, which involves flexing, abducting, and externally rotating the hip, may reproduce some pain (Fig. 6.3). Palpation of the nerve at the outlet may also reproduce the pain.

The pectineal muscle stretch (Fig. 6.4) may also indicate obturator entrapment. In this test the patient is

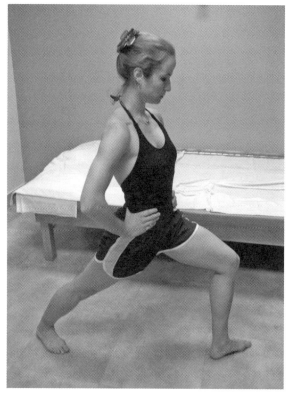

Figure 6.4   The pectineal muscle stretch.

instructed to perform a lunge with the affected leg going forward. The affected leg is also externally rotated while in this position. If pain is reproduced with this movement, it indicates a high likelihood that the patient may have obturator neuropathy.

Diagnostic Studies

Imaging studies such as MRI or radiographs are usually not needed. EMG/NCV studies can detect the presence of nerve injury. If there is still some question of the nerve injury, a diagnostic nerve block may needed.

Treatment

This is usually treated like a strain with rest, medication, and ice. If the pain continues and is refractory to conservative treatment, surgical intervention may be needed. The surgery involves separating the fascia over the pectineus and adductor muscles.

TROCHANTERIC BURSITIS

Background

The greater trochanter bursa lies between the iliotibial tract (ITB) and the greater trochanter. If the ITB is tight, friction develops and can lead to greater trochanteric bursitis. In addition, the gluteus medius attaches to the greater trochanter. If this hip abductor is weak, it affects gait biomechanics and can also lead to repetitive irritation of the bursa, resulting in bursitis. Trochanteric bursitis can also result from an acute trauma to the bursa from a fall or tackle during sporting events. This cause is less common than repetitive trauma.

Clinical Presentation

Patients characteristically complain of lateral hip pain over the greater trochanter. The pain sometimes radiates down the thigh toward the knee. Rarely the pain referral pattern may extend as far as the ankle. Patients report having increased pain at night if they try to lie on the affected side. Patients also may complain of increased pain when rising from a seated position (here, the ITB slides over the greater trochanter, causing pain). Walking and running may also exacerbate pain.

If an acute trauma precipitated the pain, the patient relates the event as immediately precipitating the pain. More often, the pain arises gradually.

Physical Examination

The hallmark finding is point tenderness over the greater trochanter that reproduces the patient's pain (Fig. 6.5). Note that if the area is tender but does not reproduce typical pain, it is not characteristic. If symptoms typically radiate down the thigh, palpation may (or sometimes may not) reproduce this symptom as well. The rest of the examination, particularly the neurologic (including

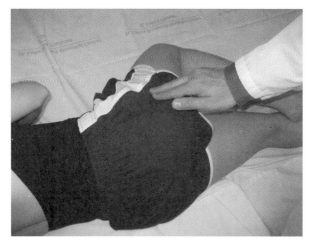

Figure 6.5 Palpation of the greater trochanter.

straight leg raise) should be negative. Sometimes, the patient has an antalgic gait, favoring the unaffected side. A full strength exam should be performed bilaterally in the lower extremities. If hip abduction is weak, it is important to try to ascertain if the weakness is secondary to pain or general weakness (from, for example, an L5 radiculopathy). This determination may be difficult if pain is limiting.

Diagnostic Studies

No diagnostic tests are routinely ordered except to exclude other potential diagnoses such as in the case of an acute trauma (e.g., to rule out fracture).

Treatment

Physical therapy, including stretching of the ITB, is very helpful for this condition. Ice is also effective for reducing inflammation in this location. Depending on the severity and duration of symptoms, a corticosteroid and anesthetic injection into the bursa can be very efficacious. These injections are not generally performed with imaging guidance. However, if ultrasound is available, it may be helpful. Otherwise, the injection should be performed at the site of maximal tenderness.

If an underlying L5 radiculopathy is suspected as a potential contributor to developing the bursitis, or if the bursitis is recurrent, it may be reasonable for the patient to have physical therapy to work on lumbar stabilization, bilateral hip strengthening, as well as addressing any muscle imbalances and/or flexibility limitations.

ILIOPSOAS TENDONITIS/BURSITIS

Background

Iliopsoas tendonitis and bursitis are closely related. Inflammation of one may readily lead to inflammation of the other. They are treated the same way and are considered together here.

Clinical Presentation

Patients typically complain of anterior hip and/or groin pain. The pain often begins insidiously and is intermittent. As the inflammation progresses, the patient notes the symptoms become more chronic. Activity, particularly any activity that involves a lot of hip flexion such as walking, running, climbing stairs, and kicking, exacerbate the symptoms. Occasionally, the pain may radiate down the anterior thigh into the knee.

Patients may also complain that their hip snaps or clicks, although snapping and clicking are not necessarily symptomatic.

Physical Examination

The classic findings on physical examination are reproduction of symptoms with resisted hip flexion and tenderness to palpation of the iliopsoas tendon as it approaches its insertion point on the lesser trochanter of the femur.

The snapping hip test can also be performed. In this test, snapping or clicking is assessed while moving a flexed, abducted, and externally rotated hip into extension. Flexing the knee may make this test easier to perform. If snapping or clicking is present, the test is considered positive for an internal "snapping hip." If pain is reproduced with this test, it suggests the presence of iliopsoas tendonitis/bursitis.

Diagnostic Studies

Radiographs may be ordered to rule out other pathology. Ultrasound can be used for diagnosis. MRI is an excellent imaging test for this disorder.

If the diagnosis is in doubt and the MRI is equivocal, too costly, or not available, injecting a local anesthetic over the iliopsoas tendonitis/bursitis may help identify it as the pain generator. Ultrasound guidance for this procedure is useful if available. If symptoms are alleviated, the diagnosis is confirmed.

Treatment

The cornerstone of treatment is rest, ice, compression, and elevation (RICE) and physical therapy. Initially, physical therapy includes gentle stretching exercises. After therapy, icing is important to help control inflammation. Therapy gradually introduces strengthening exercises, focusing on lumbar stabilization and hamstring strengthening (particularly if the patient has an anterior pelvic tilt).

A corticosteroid and anesthetic injection performed under ultrasound guidance can also be very helpful for this condition. As always, care must be used not to inject directly into the tendon.

Although rare, patients with persistent, severe symptoms despite aggressive conservative care may be surgical candidates. Surgical options include tendon lengthening, release, and partial release.

FEMORAL NECK STRESS FRACTURE

Background

Stress fractures are difficult to diagnose but important not to miss. When they are suspected, they must be pursued until the physician is satisfied it has been ruled out. Failure to do so may result in a mild stress fracture that progresses to a complete fracture, nonunion, and possibly osteonecrosis. Runners and military recruits are at particular risk for this stress fracture. The index of suspicion should also be increased for any patient who reports a recent increase in exercise intensity, and in any active woman suspected of having the female triad (amenorrhea, disordered eating, and osteoporosis).

Clinical Presentation

Patients with a femoral neck stress fracture may have vague symptoms, including deep, aching pain in the groin, buttock, and/or thigh. Patients typically (although not always) report a recent increase in their activity level. Initially, the pain is only present after strenuous activity. As the fracture progresses, pain may become more intense and limit activity. If the patient does not modify his activity level, he may begin to have pain during walking or even with minimal weightbearing.

Physical Examination

The patient may have an antalgic gait, favoring the asymptomatic side. Weightbearing on the affected leg may also be seen. Pain may be elicited with internal and external rotation of the hip. Internal rotation may be more painful than external. Log-rolling the patient may also elicit pain. Pain reproduced with a heel thump while the leg is extended is indicative of possible fracture.

If a stress fracture is suspected, care should be taken not to *over*load the extremity to prevent further progression of the fracture. Straight leg raise may also reproduce anterior thigh pain.

Diagnostic Studies

Radiographs should be obtained. If initial films are negative but suspicion remains, MRI should be obtained and the patient should be made nonweightbearing with crutches until the MRI is read. MRI is superior to bone scan for this purpose, although bone scans are often positive within 24 to 48 hours postfracture. Alternatively, if MRI is not available, the patient can remain nonweightbearing for 2 to 3 weeks and repeat radiographs can be obtained.

Treatment

For compression side (inferior medial side) nondisplaced fractures, patients typically respond well to conservative therapy. Conservative care includes nonweightbearing for approximately 3 to 4 weeks progressing to toe-touch weightbearing for an additional 2 to 3 weeks, depending on healing evidence on radiograph and pain relief. Then progression is made to full weightbearing. Weightbearing should only be done when it is pain free. Physical therapy should also be performed, focusing on stretching and progressive strengthening once weightbearing is resumed. Patients may expect to return to their sport within 3 months.

Displaced compression fractures in young patients are considered a surgical emergency.

For tension side (superior, often transverse orientation) fractures, some physicians advocate surgery for displaced *and* nondisplaced fractures. Others advocate surgical pinning only for displaced tension side fractures.

If the female triad is suspected, patients should receive appropriate nutritional and psychological support and appropriate referrals.

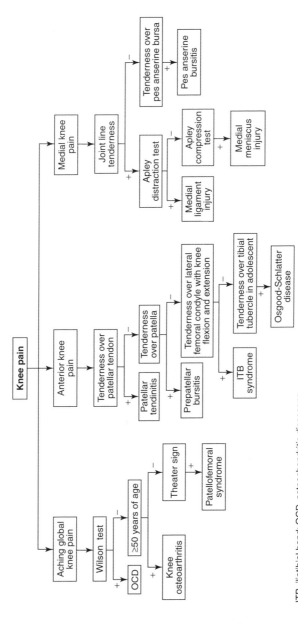

ITB, iliotibial band; OCD, osteochondritis dissecans.

Knee Pain

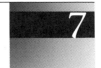

Red Flag Signs and Symptoms

Any of these signs and symptoms should prompt urgent evaluation and appropriate intervention:

Fevers
Chills
Hot, swollen joint
Progressive neurologic symptoms
Loss of pulses

KNEE OSTEOARTHRITIS

Background

Knee osteoarthritis (OA) is a very common cause of knee pain, particularly in patients older than 55 years with knee pain. The prevalence increases with increasing age. The medial compartment (including the medial tibial plateau and medial femoral condyle) of the knee is most often affected. Obesity, history of knee injury, and quadriceps weakness all increase the likelihood of developing knee OA.

Clinical Presentation

Patients are typically older than 55 years and complain of insidious onset of knee pain. The medial side, or anterior and medial side, of the knee may be most painful; however, the whole knee is also often painful. The pain is often described as dull and aching. Initially, the pain is present only with activities such as ascending and descending stairs (particularly going down stairs).

As the disease progresses, the pain becomes present with less strenuous activities such as walking long distances. The knee also becomes stiff and the patient may note that it swells up after use. Patients may report that it takes "a little while to get going" after standing up and walking or after waking up in the morning. As the patient walks, the knee warms up and feels better. However, if the patient walks "too much," the pain is exacerbated and limits walking.

Patients may also complain of locking, catching, or stiffness, particularly after prolonged sitting.

As the disease becomes more severe, pain may be present at night or even wake the patient from sleep.

Physical Examination

The patient may have an antalgic gait, favoring the asymptomatic side. A mild effusion may be present, although a hot and swollen knee should raise suspicion for a septic knee. Crepitus may be noted with passive extension and flexion of the knee. The joint line may be tender. However, there is not typically one tender point that reproduces the patient's symptoms. Rather, knee OA produces more diffuse symptoms than that. Comparison with the asymptomatic side may reveal mild quadriceps atrophy.

Diagnostic Studies

Radiographs should be obtained (Fig. 7.1). Importantly, severity of OA on radiograph does not necessarily correlate with degree of symptoms. Characteristic findings include asymmetric joint space narrowing, osteophytes, subchondral cysts, and other findings of OA. Medial joint line often reveals most of the OA; however, a tunnel view may also reveal osteophytes and other OA findings. The lateral side often has findings of OA but not as pronounced as the medial side.

If a septic knee is suspected, arthrocentesis should be performed and the appropriate labs (cell count, crystals, glucose, Gram stain, culture, protein) sent.

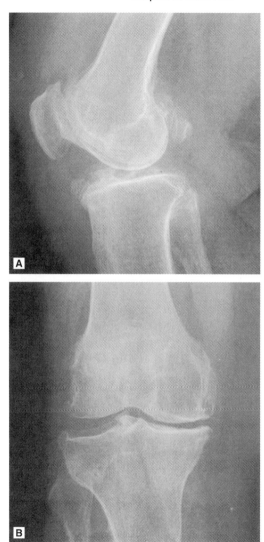

Figure 7.1   Radiograph of knee osteoarthritis. (From Moskowitz et al. *Osteoarthritis Diagnosis and Medical/Surgical Management.* 4th ed. Philadelphia, Pa: Lippincott Williams & Wilkins, 2007, with permission.)

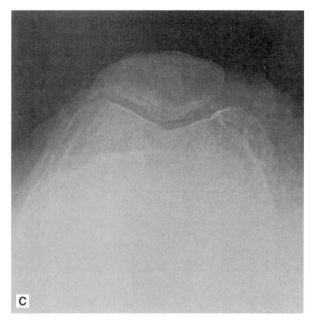

Figure 7.1 *(continued)*

Treatment

The cornerstone of treatment, physical therapy that emphasizes strengthening of the quadriceps, should be started. Closed-chain exercises (foot is fixed, as in a leg press) may be preferable for this purpose because they have less sheer forces than open-chain exercises (foot is not fixed, as in knee extension). Gait biomechanics should also be addressed with therapy.

Importantly, the patient needs to continue to be active. Once the knee is painful, the tendency is to stay off the knee. However, in OA, the cartilage is degraded. To continue to provide nourishment to the remaining cartilage, weightbearing and movement are essential. If the patient stays off the painful extremity, the remaining cartilage quickly erodes and the process is very hard to address non-surgically. Of course, the patient should not work through too much pain. A healthy balance must be reached.

Nonsteroidal anti-inflammatory drugs (NSAIDs) and acetaminophen may be helpful as pain relievers.

Oral supplementation with glucosamine and chondroitin sulfate may also be helpful, although more research is needed to make definitive recommendations. An advantage of these supplements is that they appear to not have the same negative side-effect profile as NSAIDs.

An intra-articular injection of steroid and anesthetic is very helpful in reducing symptoms (Fig. 7.2). This is often done blind, although it can also be done under ultrasound or fluoroscopic guidance to ensure optimal placement. These injections typically provide 4 months to 1 year of relief. They may be repeated up to three times yearly as needed. As the disease progresses, the steroid injections tend to become less effective.

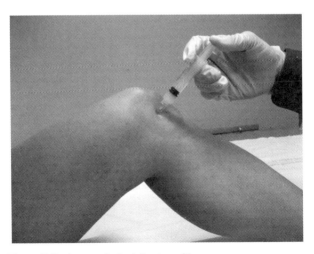

Figure 7.2   Intra-articular injection of knee.

INTRA-ARTICULAR KNEE INJECTION

There are multiple approaches to the knee joint. An intra-articular injection can be performed via lateral, inferolateral, inferomedial, superolateral, or superomedial routes. Every knee is different, and some knees may predispose to being injected from different directions depending on the anatomy. In general, the authors of this book favor an inferomedial approach.

Informed consent is first obtained. The patient lies supine with the knee flexed to about 30 to 45 degrees so the foot is flat on the examination table. The physician runs hands superiorly along the tibia until the fingers fall off the tibial plateau on the medial side of the patella. This point is marked. The authors favor using a 25-gauge, 1.5 inch needle, 40 mg of triamcinolone acetate, and 4 mL of 1% lidocaine. Sterilize the marked spot using three iodine swabs and an alcohol pad. Using sterile technique, aim the needle parallel to the ground directly into the joint. Straight ahead, the needle runs into the femoral condyle. Gently touch bone and then back off the bone. Always aspirate before injecting. If blood is found in the aspirate, reposition. There should be no aspirate in this injection. If an effusion is present in the knee, then an aspiration should be done first. See the next paragraph for details on how to perform an aspiration. When there is no aspirate and the injectate flows smoothly, inject. Clean the iodine off with alcohol pads.

If an effusion is present, it should be aspirated from the joint cavity. Aspiration helps provide symptom relief. There are multiple ways to approach aspiration. The one favored by the authors involves using a 22-gauge, 1.5 inch needle and inserting into the joint. For this injection, an anesthetic spray should be used. The joint is then aspirated. The syringe is switched with the needle still in the joint. The new syringe contains the injectate (40 mg of triamcinolone acetate and 4 mL of 1% lidocaine), which is injected. Extension tubing can be used to facilitate an easier transfer of syringes.

Intra-articular injections of hyaluronic acid are also very effective for certain patients with knee OA. Ideally, these injections should be performed on patients with mild to moderate knee OA. They are less effective once the OA is severe. The hyaluronic acid injections are usually given once per week for 3 to 5 weeks depending on the preparation used. They may need to be repeated once every 6 months.

When aggressive conservative measures fail, several surgical options, including arthroscopy and osteotomy, are available. The most common and most effective surgical treatment is total knee arthroplasty. In the right patient population, this procedure greatly increases quality of life after surgery.

MENISCUS TEAR

Background

The menisci are fibrocartilaginous pads that serve as shock absorbers for the knee joint. The medial meniscus is more crescent shaped, and the lateral meniscus more circular. Only the periphery of the menisci (outer third) receives blood supply. A tear in this zone is said to be a "red" tear. A tear in the center two-thirds is said to be a "white" tear. Red tears are much more likely to heal with conservative care.

Clinical Presentation

Two typical types of patients present with meniscal tears: younger patients with acute pain and older patients with degenerative tears that occur gradually.

Younger patients are generally younger than 50 years. They report a history of an acute injury, such as a twisting injury with the knee in flexed position. This may occur, for example, during pivoting in basketball or soccer. Following the injury, patients report onset of pain, swelling, and/or stiffness. Sometimes, the pain begins immediately after the injury. Other times, the patient may not notice the pain until later that night. Patients may complain of "locking," or "catching." Weightbearing, getting up from a seated position, and ascending stairs may exacerbate symptoms. Mild swelling generally occurs the day after the injury. Patients may localize their pain to the medial or lateral aspect of the knee. Occasionally, they may have difficulty identifying the exact location of their pain.

Older patients are generally older than 50 years. They typically present with an insidious onset of symptoms. Sometimes they recall a history of trauma to the knee (e.g., twisting). However, the injury does not immediately precipitate symptoms. Symptoms may include pain, locking, catching, and/or giving way.

Physical Examination

An effusion may be present on examination. Classic findings include joint line tenderness that reproduces the patient's symptoms. The McMurray test and Apley compression and distraction test are very useful for assessing meniscal injuries. In the McMurray test (Fig. 7.3), the patient lies

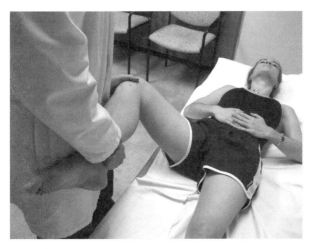

Figure 7.3 McMurray test.

supine with hip and knee fully flexed. The physician then externally rotates the tibia and applies a valgus force while extending the knee to assess the medial meniscus. To assess the lateral meniscus, the physician internally rotates the tibia and applies a varus force while extending the knee. A palpable snap or click is indicative of a meniscal tear.

In Apley's compression and distraction test (Figs. 7.4A and B), the patient lies prone with the knee flexed to 90 degrees. The physician stabilizes the patient's thigh with one hand and with the other hand internally and externally rotates the patient's tibia while applying a compressive force (driving the patients tibia *into* the table). The physician then applies a traction force to the tibia

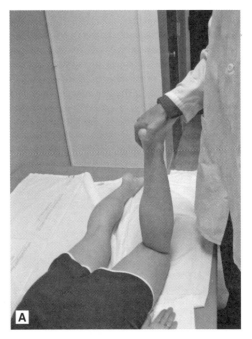

Figure 7.4   (A) Apley compression.

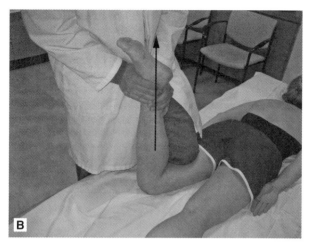

Figure 7.4 (*continued*)   **(B)** Distraction test.

(pulling the tibia *off* the table). If the patient has reproduction of symptoms with compressive internal and
external rotation but not with traction, this indicates a
meniscal injury. If symptoms are reproduced with traction, however, this may indicate a ligamentous injury
because in traction, the menisci are *unloaded* and should
not cause pain.

Patients with suspected menisci injuries should also
be interrogated for ligamentous instability. Anterior cruciate ligament (ACL) injuries in particular commonly
occur with acute medial meniscal tears.

Diagnostic Studies

Radiographs should be obtained to rule out bony
abnormality.

Magnetic resonance imaging (MRI) can be obtained
to confirm the diagnosis if it is in doubt. MRI can also
aid in prognostication based on the size, type, and location of the tear. Also, if surgery is being considered, MRI
should be obtained.

Treatment

Acute injuries may be treated initially with protection, rest, ice, compression, and elevation (PRICE). If symptoms persist for 1 to 2 weeks and are not improving, physical therapy that focuses on early range of motion and progressing to strengthening exercises of the quadriceps and hamstrings is effective. Quadriceps strengthening should begin with closed-chain exercises. If an effusion is present and significant, aspiration may alleviate symptoms. Although controversial, some physicians advocate an injection of corticosteroid and anesthetic into the joint if it is resistant to 4 to 6 weeks of conservative care.

Degenerative, chronic tears are likewise treated with physical therapy initially.

Patients with tears in the "white" avascular center of the meniscus may require early surgical intervention. In addition, patients with bucket-handle tears may require surgery. As with other conditions, severe, debilitating symptoms may require earlier surgical intervention. The risks of postponing surgery include the possibility that the tear will expand. Of course, surgery also carries risks, including the possibility of increasing the likelihood of future osteoarthritis. Arthroscopic surgical options include partial meniscectomy and/or repair.

LIGAMENT INJURY

Background

The ACL, posterior cruciate ligament (PCL), medial collateral ligament (MCL), and lateral collateral ligament (LCL) all provide support to the knee. Injury patterns follow fairly predictable patterns. ACL injuries result from a hyperextension or twisting injury. ACL injuries frequently occur in combination with a medial meniscal injury. MCL injuries follow a valgus force without rotation. LCL injuries follow a varus force. PCL injuries are less common but typically result following a car accident in which the knee hits the dashboard or a pure hyperflexion injury to the knee. The injury can occur in combination with another injury such as an ACL tear.

Clinical Presentation

Patients typically report a specific injury during an athletic event. Patients may report an audible "pop" at the time of injury. Pain and swelling typically occur and worsen as the day progresses after the injury.

Following an ACL tear, patients may report instability. PCL tears also may result in a feeling of instability in the knee.

Instability is not common after an isolated sprain of the MCL or LCL.

Physical Examination

Ecchymosis and an effusion may be present on examination. Range of motion is often limited.

The classic findings include interrogation for stability of the ligament. With all of these tests, the asymptomatic side should be compared with the symptomatic one. A lax endpoint on the symptomatic side compared with the asymptomatic one indicates a positive test.

The ACL is assessed with the Lachman test and the anterior drawer test. The Lachman test (Fig. 7.5) is more sensitive for an ACL tear. In this test, the patient's knee is flexed to 20 to 30 degrees. The physician stabilizes the patient's femur with one hand and pulls the tibia anteriorly with the other hand.

In the anterior drawer test (Fig. 7.6), the physician flexes the patient's knee to 90 degrees and sits on the patient's foot, stabilizing it. The physician then cups hands behind the patient's upper calf and pulls the tibia toward the physician.

The MCL and LCL are assessed by applying a valgus and varus stress, respectively, with the knee in 20 degrees of flexion (to relax the joint capsule) and also in full extension.

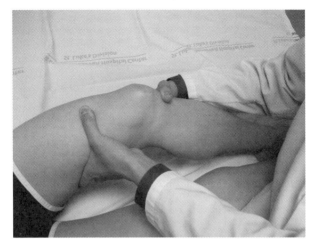

Figure 7.5   Lachman test

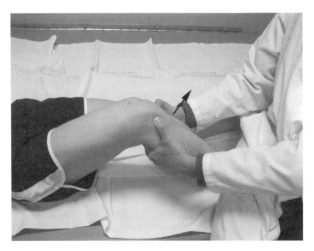

Figure 7.6   Anterior drawer test.

The PCL is assessed with the posterior drawer test. In this test, the patient lies supine with the knee at 90 degrees of flexion. The physician sits on the foot, stabilizing it, and pushes the tibia posteriorly.

The ligaments should also be palpated for tenderness, which is often present (except in the case of a PCL tear).

Diagnostic Studies

Radiographs should be obtained to rule out bony abnormality, particularly an avulsion fracture.

MRI is not routinely indicated but may be helpful to confirm the diagnosis and help rule out associated injury. Also, if surgery is being considered, MRI is indicated.

Treatment

If a large effusion is present, aspiration is helpful to relieve pain.

Patients with an ACL injury should initially be treated with PRICE. Early range-of-motion exercises are begun. A structured physical therapy program is very helpful that focuses on flexibility and strengthening of the surrounding musculature. The decision of whether to have surgery is based on the extent of injury, other injuries present, and the patient's level of functioning and expectations. If the patient is a competitive athlete who wants to return to competition, surgery may be needed. For older patients, or patients wishing to avoid surgery because of comorbidities, functional bracing may be helpful.

Patients with isolated MCL tears are typically treated conservatively with PRICE, crutches, and/or bracing if needed, and physical therapy.

Patients with LCL tears are treated nonsurgically except for grade III tears that typically require surgical intervention.

Patients with PCL tears typically have associated injuries, and treatment needs to take these into account. In patients with isolated PCL tears, PRICE and physical therapy are generally sufficient treatment.

PATELLOFEMORAL SYNDROME

Background

Patellofemoral syndrome (PFS) is characterized by a constellation of symptoms and pathologies. The term *chondromalacia* historically was used to describe this syndrome. However, chondromalacia refers to pathologic changes being present on the articular surface of the patella, which may or may not be present. The exact causes and pathologic mechanisms of PFS remain somewhat controversial. Anatomic misalignment of the patella was thought to play a primary role. Although patella alignment may be an important feature in some patients, other factors, such as quadriceps weakness and patella overload, are believed to be equally or more important in other patients.

Clinical Presentation

Patients are typically younger than 45 years (although they can be older). Patients complain of anterior knee pain that is worse with weightbearing activities. Patients often report pain after prolonged sitting (known as the positive theater sign). Some patients only note symptoms initially with intensive exercise such as doing squats in the gym, climbing stairs, or running. Other patients only note symptoms *after* completing vigorous activity. If these symptoms are not addressed, they tend to worsen. Less commonly, patients may complain of locking or catching.

Physical Examination

On examination, an effusion is typically *not* present.

An increased Q-angle and laterally tracking patella may be present. The Q-angle is measured with the patient seated and the knee fully extended. An imaginary line is drawn from the anterior superior iliac spine to the center of the patella. A second line is drawn from above the center of the patella down to the tibial tuberosity. The superior

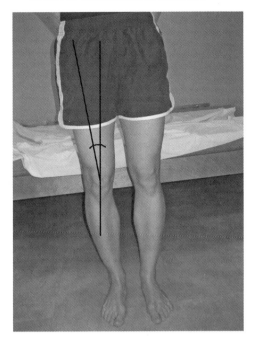

Figure 7.7   Q-angle.

angle created by the intersection of these lines is the Q-angle (Fig. 7.7). In males, a normal Q-angle is 10 to 15 degrees. In females, it may be up to 20 degrees. If the Q-angle is increased, or if the patella laterally tracks during knee extension and flexion, misalignment of the patella may need to be addressed.

Another good test for PFS is to have the patient lie supine and palpate the undersurface of the patella. Patients with PFS typically have pain with this maneuver.

Diagnostic Studies

Radiographs are not routinely obtained but may help rule out other conditions such as OA.

Treatment

The cornerstone of treatment for PFS is ice and physical therapy. Physical therapy should focus on quadriceps strengthening using closed-chain kinetic exercises such as modified squats. Straight leg raises also are appropriate. Stretching should focus on the quadriceps, hamstrings, and iliotibial band.

McConnell taping may also be helpful for some patients. An infrapatellar strap may be used, particularly during athletic activities.

Surgical intervention is not generally required, but options include patellar resurfacing and lateral release.

ILIOTIBIAL BAND SYNDROME

Background

The iliotibial band (ITB) is a dense fibrous band of tissue that arises from the anterior superior iliac spine and runs inferiorly along the lateral surface of the thigh, crossing the knee and attaching the Gerdy tubercle on the lateral tibia. During knee extension and flexion, the ITB glides over the lateral femoral condyle (proximal to the knee).

Clinical Presentation

Patients typically participate in activities that involve repetitive knee flexion and extension. It is most commonly seen in long-distance runners (some physicians call this syndrome "runner's knee"). Patients complain of anterior-lateral knee pain that is exacerbated by running. Heel strike, in particular, may be painful. Climbing stairs also may be more painful. An audible popping may be present in the knee with walking and/or running.

Physical Examination

On examination, tenderness to palpation over the lateral femoral condyle is characteristic. The point tenderness may be more pronounced while flexing and extending the knee.

Diagnostic Studies

None are routinely ordered.

Treatment

Ice, relative rest, and physical therapy that focuses on stretching the ITB is first-line treatment. Modalities and soft tissue mobilization may be helpful during physical therapy in the acutely painful period. Patients who have persistent pain despite conservative care may respond well to a steroid and anesthetic injection at the point of maximal tenderness. Orthotics may also be needed to correct excessive pronation if present.

Recurrent ITB syndrome needs further investigation to determine any biomechanical factors that may be contributing. The patient's offending activity (e.g., running) should be investigated. The patient may need to alter his or her running stride.

PATELLA TENDONITIS (JUMPER'S KNEE)

Background

Patella tendonitis is typically an overuse injury of the knee extensor muscles. Patients often participate in jumping or kicking sports. The patella tendon inserts into the tibial tuberosity and enables the quadriceps to extend the lower leg.

Clinical Presentation

Patients are typically younger than 40 years and present with anterior knee pain. The pain is exacerbated by stair climbing, squatting, and participating in sports such as soccer, volleyball, basketball, or track.

Physical Examination

The hallmark examination finding is point tenderness over the quadriceps tendon that reproduces the patient's symptoms. Resisted knee extension may also reproduce symptoms.

Diagnostic Studies

None are routinely indicated.

Treatment

Relative rest, ice, and physical therapy form the cornerstone of treatment. Physical therapy utilizes modalities, soft tissue mobilization, and stretching and strengthening exercises. NSAIDs and topical analgesic creams are often helpful, particularly in the acute phase of the injury.

Steroid injections are not advised because they may lead to tendon rupture. The knee should not be immobilized because further stiffening of the joint and atrophy of the muscles may result.

PES ANSERINE BURSITIS

Background

The pes anserinus marks the location where three tendons attach to the medial knee. These tendons are the sartorius, gracilis, and semitendinosus, and they can be remembered by the mnemonic "Say grace before tea." The bursa covering this location has a tendency to become inflamed, particularly in patients with diabetes and in patients with a history of MCL injury and/or early medial OA. Obesity also increases the risk of pes anserine bursitis.

Clinical Presentation

Patients typically report medial knee pain over the pes anserine bursa. Pain may be exacerbated with climbing

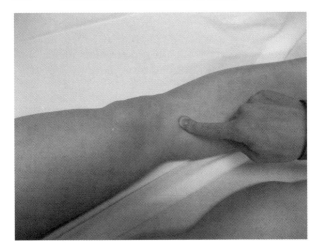

Figure 7.8   Pes anserine palpation.

stairs. Patients may note swelling over the bursa; however, swelling is less common than in other locations for bursitis.

Physical Examination

Point tenderness over the pes anserine, which is approximately 2 inches inferior to the anteromedial joint line (Fig. 7.8), is the classic finding. An effusion in this location may also be present.

Diagnostic Studies

None are routinely ordered. If pain has been chronic, radiographs may be obtained to rule out bony abnormality.

Treatment

The cornerstone of treatment is ice, topical analgesics, and correcting any muscle imbalances with physical

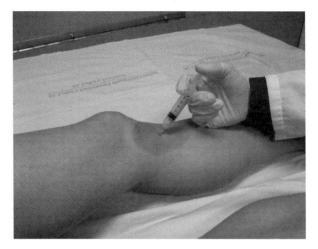

Figure 7.9   Pes anserine injection.

therapy. An intrabursal injection of steroid and anesthetic is helpful for resistant or severe cases (Fig. 7.9). This may be done under ultrasound guidance for optimal needle placement or injected at the site of maximal tenderness. As always, care must be taken to not inject directly into a tendon. If an effusion is present, aspiration should be performed first, and if the fluid appears septic, it should be sent for appropriate studies and steroids should then *not* be injected until sepsis is ruled out.

PES ANSERINE BURSA INJECTION

After informed consent is obtained, identify point of maximal tenderness over the pes anserine bursa. The authors favor using a 25-gauge, 1.5 inch needle, 40 mg of triamcinolone acetate, and 2 mL of 1% lidocaine. Mark the spot of maximal tenderness. Sterilize this area using three iodine swabs and an alcohol pad. Using sterile technique, aim the needle perpendicular to the marked spot. Always aspirate before injecting. If blood is found in the aspirate, reposition. If there is an aspirate, it should not be bloody. When there is no aspirate and the injectate flows smoothly, inject. Clean the iodine off with alcohol pads. If an effusion is present, aspirate first using a 22-gauge, 1.5 inch needle and an empty syringe. Then switch the syringe to the syringe filled with injectate and inject it.

PREPATELLAR BURSITIS (HOUSEMAID'S KNEE)

Background

A bursa is located between the patella and the skin. In patients who spend a lot of time kneeling (e.g., maids), this bursa can become inflamed. It is important to consider sepsis as a possible cause of the bursitis so it is not missed.

Clinical Presentation

Patients may report a history of repetitive kneeling or having fallen on their knee. Patients complain of anterior knee pain. They may also complain of swelling and redness. Walking and climbing stairs may exacerbate symptoms. Kneeling on the knee is particularly painful.

Physical Examination

The classic finding is tenderness over the prepatellar bursa. Swelling and warmth may also be noted and should prompt increased suspicion for septic bursitis.

Diagnostic Studies

None are routinely indicated. However, a low threshold of clinical suspicion should be kept for septic bursitis.

If septic bursitis is suspected, the bursal fluid should be aspirated and sent for appropriate studies (e.g., Gram stain, culture, white blood cell count).

Treatment

Septic bursitis can be treated with appropriate antibiotics orally, if mild, or intravenously if severe. Common pathogens include *Staphylococcus aureus* and *Streptococcus*. These pathogens can be treated empirically and then the antibiotics altered depending on the results of the fluid culture and sensitivity.

Nonseptic prepatellar bursitis responds well to ice, topical analgesics, and physical therapy. An injection of steroid and anesthetic can also be very helpful.

OSTEOCHONDRITIS DISSECANS

Background

In osteochondritis dissecans (OCD), an osteochondral fragment separates from the articular surface. The underlying bone maintains its vascularity, distinguishing OCD from osteonecrosis in which the vascularity of the underlying bone is compromised. In the knee, OCD occurs most commonly on the posterolateral aspect of the medial femoral condyle. OCD in the knee is thought to be mostly caused by repetitive trauma during tibial internal rotation between the tibia and lateral aspect of the medial femoral condyle.

Clinical Presentation

Patients typically present with poorly defined, aching pain in the knee. The symptoms typically have an insidious onset. As the symptoms progress, the pain may become more constant and patients may also complain of catching and/or locking of the knee. Catching and/or locking generally indicate a severe lesion that has progressed to a loose body.

Physical Examination

An effusion may or may not be present. With the knee flexed to 90 degrees, palpation of the medial femoral condyle often reveals tenderness. The Wilson test should be performed. In this test, the patient lies supine and hip and knee are passively flexed to 90 degrees. The test is positive when the patient has pain with the knee internally rotated at 20 to 30 degrees of extension and no pain when the knee is externally rotated. Of note, this test only identifies OCD of the medial femoral condyle (which is where it occurs in the knee about 80% of the time).

Diagnostic Studies

Radiographs should be obtained and may reveal the OCD lesion as a lucency. MRI with contrast should also be obtained, particularly if surgical intervention is being considered.

Treatment

Treatment depends on the stage of the lesion and the skeletal maturity of the patient. Skeletally immature patients (e.g., girls younger than 11 years, boys younger than 13 years) tend to heal adequately with nonoperative care. However, if symptoms persist despite conservative care for >6 months, or if loose bodies are present, surgical intervention should be strongly considered. If skeletal maturity has been reached but the lesion is small, stable, and vascularized, nonsurgical care may be appropriate. Nonsurgical care includes activity modification so that the knee is not painful during activities, crutches if needed, ice, and sometimes a knee immobilizer.

Patients who have reached skeletal maturity and have a large, unstable, avascular lesion often respond better to surgery; however, this decision is made clinically based on symptoms as well as anatomy. There are many surgical options including arthroscopic subchondral drilling, fixation with bone pegs, autologous chondrocyte transplantation, and autologous osteochondral mosaic-plasty. Patients should discuss all the risks and benefits of these procedures with their potential surgeon.

OSGOOD-SCHLATTER DISEASE

Background

Osgood-Schlatter is one of the most common causes of anterior knee pain in active adolescents between 8 and 15 years of age. It is believed to be essentially a traction injury of the cartilage at the secondary ossification center of the tibial tubercle where the patella tendon inserts that results from repetitive knee extension leading to subacute stress fractures.

Clinical Presentation

Patients are typically between 8 and 15 years of age and complain of anterior knee pain that is worse with activity such as running and jumping. Patients typically report participation in an athletic activity such as soccer, dance, football, basketball, volleyball, or gymnastics. The symptoms often develop gradually and worsen over time.

Physical Examination

The hallmark examination finding is point tenderness over the tibial tubercle (Fig. 7.10). Swelling over the tubercle may also be present.

Diagnostic Studies

Radiographs should be obtained. These films may be normal or may show changes consistent with soft tissue swelling. Severe cases may reveal radiodense fragmentation of the tibial tubercle. MRI may be obtained but is not routinely ordered.

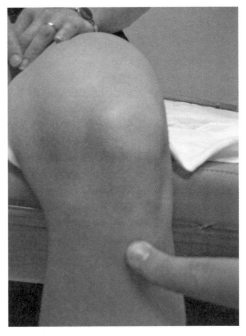

Figure 7.10   Pain over the tibial tubercle in Osgood-Schlatter disease.

Treatment

Education and activity modification are the most important points of treatment. Activities should be limited to those that are not painful. Ice should be applied after activity for 4 to 8 weeks, even if the activity was not painful. Physical therapy may be helpful and should emphasize stretching the quadriceps, hamstrings, and iliotibial band. A knee brace can be used to help facilitate return to sports after 6 to 8 weeks of relative rest.

Rarely, if symptoms persist despite rest and conservative care, surgical removal of the painful fragmented ossified portion of the tubercle may be required.

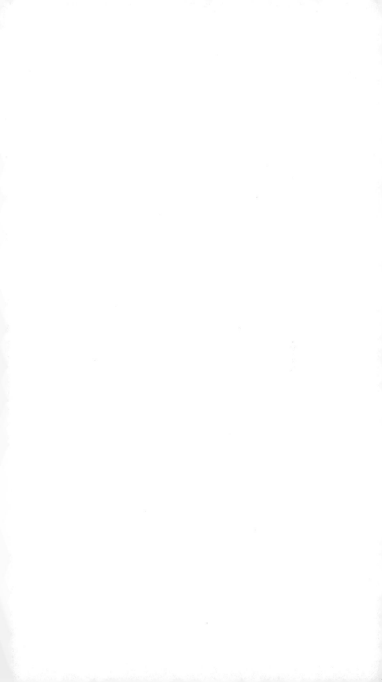

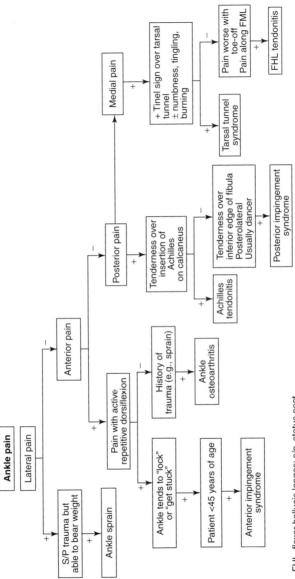

FHL, flexor hallucis longos; s/p, status post.

Ankle and Foot Pain

Red Flag Signs and Symptoms

Any of these signs and symptoms should prompt urgent evaluation and appropriate intervention:

Fevers
Chills
Hot, swollen joint
Progressive neurologic symptoms
Loss of pulses

ANKLE SPRAIN

Background

Ankle sprains are a very common musculoskeletal problem and account for approximately 75% of injuries to the ankle. They are the most common injury in athletics overall, and they are also relatively common in the general population. The anterior talofibular ligament (ATFL) is the most commonly injured ligament. The calcaneofibular ligament (CFL) is the second most common. The posterior talofibular ligament is only injured in severe sprains.

A grade I sprain indicates a stretching of the ATFL and often also the CFL. A grade II sprain indicates a partial tearing of the ATFL and stretching of the CFL. A grade III sprain indicates a full tearing of the ATFL and CFL and a partial tearing of the PTFL.

The medial deltoid ligament is a strong, dense structure that is rarely injured.

It is important to diagnose and treat ankle sprains appropriately to help prevent chronic ankle instability and pain.

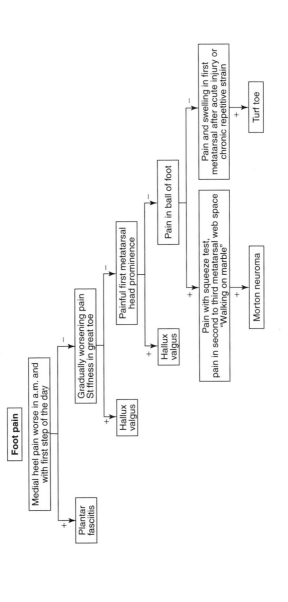

Foot pain

Medial heel pain worse in a.m. and with first step of the day
- **+** → Plantar fasciitis
- **–** → Gradually worsening pain Stiffness in great toe
  - **+** → Hallux valgus
  - **–** → Painful first metatarsal head prominence
    - **+** → Hallux valgus
    - **–** → Pain in ball of foot
      - **+** → Pain with squeeze test, pain in second to third metatarsal web space "Walking on marble"
        - **+** → Morton neuroma
      - **–** → Pain and swelling in first metatarsal after acute injury or chronic repetitive strain
        - **+** → Turf toe

Clinical Presentation

Patients generally report an injury in which they "fell over" their foot. On specific questioning, the patient reports the ankle having been in plantar flexion and inversion in the injury. For example, patients may state that they "stumbled over" an inverted foot. At the time of the injury, some patients report hearing a "pop."

Patients report pain over their lateral ankle. Often, the patient also reports swelling. Weightbearing is difficult (grade I or II) or not possible (grade III) after the injury.

Physical Examination

On examination, ecchymosis and swelling may be present. The involved ligaments are tender. Assess if the patient is able to weight-bear on the involved ankle and how many steps the patient is able to take.

Palpate the medial and lateral malleoli, foot, and fibula and tibia along their entire course.

The anterior drawer and talar tilt test should be performed. In the anterior drawer test (Fig. 8.1), the physician stabilizes the ankle in 20 degrees of plantarflexion with

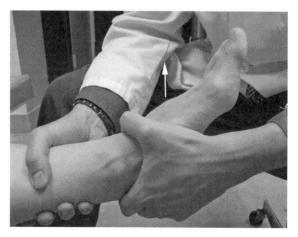

Figure 8.1   Ankle anterior drawer test.

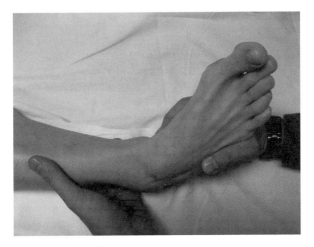

Figure 8.2   Talar tilt test.

one hand and with the other hand pulls the calcaneus anteriorly. Excessive anteroposterior glide (in comparison with the asymptomatic side) is considered a positive test and indicates an injury to the ATFL.

In the talar tilt test (Fig. 8.2), the physician inverts the ankle and compares the laxity of the asymptomatic and symptomatic sides. Increased laxity is considered a positive test and indicates an injury to the CFL.

Diagnostic Studies

The Ottawa ankle rules were developed to help determine which patients with ankle injuries should get radiographs and which ones do not need them. According to a slightly modified version of these rules, if the patient presents within 10 days of injury and is able to bear weight for four steps on the injured ankle *and* does not have any tenderness in the following areas then the patient does not require radiographs:

Medial and lateral malleoli
Base of the fifth metatarsal
Navicular bone
Posterior inferior 4 inches of the fibula and tibia

If the patient is not able to bear weight on the injured ankle or has pain in any of the areas just listed, however, ankle radiographs, including anteroposterior, lateral, and mortise views, are indicated.

In addition, foot tenderness reveals the need for foot radiographs to rule out a possible concomitant fracture.

Magnetic resonance imaging (MRI) is not routinely indicated. However, if symptoms persist for >6 weeks despite aggressive conservative care, MRI should be considered for further evaluation.

Treatment

First-line treatment for grade I and II sprains includes protection, rest, ice, compression, and elevation (PRICE). Nonsteroidal anti-inflammatory drugs (NSAIDs) can also be taken. Weightbearing should be performed as tolerated. Crutches may be required initially. An air stirrup, brace, or ankle taping is also helpful at first. Patients should return to full gait as tolerated when it is pain free.

Physical therapy is essential and should emphasize early range of motion exercises progressing to proprioceptive and strengthening exercises. Failure to participate fully in an active therapy program may lead to subsequent chronic pain and/or ankle instability.

Patients may return to sport when they can run, jump 10 times on the injured foot, stand for 1 minute on the injured foot with their eyes closed, and pivot on the injured foot without pain.

Patients with a grade III sprain who participate in athletic activities or those who have associated fractures may require surgical intervention.

ACHILLES TENDONITIS (RETROCALCANEAL BURSITIS; HAGLUND SYNDROME)

Background

In the posterior heel, where the Achilles tendon inserts on the calcaneus, are several structures that can cause pain.

The tendon can become fibrotic (tendinosis) and/or inflamed (tendonitis). There is a bursa between the tendon and the skin (pre-Achilles bursa) and a bursa between the tendon and the calcaneus (retrocalcaneal bursa). Both of these bursae can become inflamed (bursitis). In Haglund syndrome, the calcaneus impinges on the Achilles tendon (usually because of a benign overgrowth of the calcaneus, termed the *Haglund deformity*) and results in Achilles tendonitis *and* retrocalcaneal bursitis. Even without a Haglund deformity, any of the conditions just described may coexist. Because they are treated very similarly, they are discussed here together.

When younger patients (between 10 and 14 years of age) complain of posterior heel pain, they may have Sever disease. This is believed to be an overuse injury in the setting of a tight Achilles tendon, which results in a retrocalcaneal apophysitis (where the Achilles tendon attaches to the calcaneus).

Clinical Presentation

Patients typically complain of posterior heel pain (anywhere from 2 inches above the calcaneus to the calcaneus) that is exacerbated by activities such as walking and running. Often, women report wearing high-heeled shoes. In children, the pain typically begins at the beginning of a new sport season.

Physical Examination

The hallmark examination finding is tenderness over, around, or immediately anterior to the Achilles tendon as it inserts on the calcaneus. The Achilles tendon is also often found to be tight. A small effusion may be present.

Diagnostic Studies

Radiographs may be ordered to rule out bony abnormality, including the Haglund deformity. In older patients, calcifications of the Achilles tendon may be seen.

Treatment

Rest, ice, compression, and elevation (RICE) is the corner-stone of initial treatment. Activities should be modified so they are not painful. A heel lift may be used temporarily to minimize pressure. Importantly, the patient should begin a physical therapy program that emphasizes stretching the Achilles tendon. Occasionally, casting may be used to reduce movement of the tendon. NSAIDs may also be helpful.

Injections should not be performed in this area because of the risk of rupturing the Achilles tendon.

In the case of the Haglund deformity, surgical excision of the bony overgrowth may be required in patients who do not respond to more conservative therapy.

Sever disease is also treated conservatively. Patients usually respond well to RICE and physical therapy. Patients can return to sports once they are pain free and have improved their ankle flexibility. They should continue an Achilles stretching program and icing to help prevent further problems once back at athletics.

ANKLE OSTEOARTHRITIS

Background

Patients with ankle osteoarthritis (OA) typically have a history of trauma to the ankle joint. Ankle OA in general is not as common as OA in other areas of the body. If a history of trauma is not present, rheumatoid arthritis should be more expected.

Clinical Presentation

Patients typically present with gradually increasing pain in the ankle joint. On questioning, they usually relate a history of ankle trauma that may have occurred in the distant past. Patients may also complain of ankle stiffness and swelling. The pain is typically primarily in the anterior ankle. Weightbearing exacerbates the pain.

Physical Examination

Patients may walk with an antalgic gait in which they favor the unaffected side. A mild effusion of the ankle may be present. Passive range of motion may reproduce pain. Range of motion is also often reduced.

Diagnostic Studies

Weightbearing radiographs should be obtained.

Treatment

RICE, physical therapy, and NSAIDs are appropriate first-line treatment for ankle OA. In addition, an intra-articular steroid injection, preferably performed under ultrasound or fluoroscopic guidance, can be very helpful.

Research is promising but still ongoing into the potential use of intra-articular hyaluronic acid injections for ankle OA.

Occasionally, an ankle-foot orthosis (AFO) can be used to allow the ankle joint to rest after an acute flare-up of OA. However, if an AFO is used, exercises should be continued to maintain flexibility within the joint.

When aggressive conservative care is insufficient, surgical options include ankle arthrodesis and total ankle replacement.

TARSAL TUNNEL SYNDROME

Background

The tarsal tunnel is located posterior to the medial malleolus. Through it pass the posterior tibial nerve, posterior tibial artery, and tendons of the tibialis posterior, flexor digitorum longus, and flexor hallucis longus. The mnemonic "Tom, Dick, and Harry" is sometimes used to remember these structures.

Compression of the posterior tibial nerve within the tarsal tunnel can occur as a result of biomechanical causes, a ganglion, bony lesion, trauma, or idiopathic reasons.

Clinical Presentation

Patients typically present with vague symptoms of diffuse medial ankle pain. Paresthesias, including burning, tingling, and/or numbness, commonly occur over the medial ankle over the tunnel and radiate into the arch of the foot. Patients generally report that the symptoms are worse with running and other activities and better with rest. Nighttime pain is also not uncommon. Occasionally, the pain and paresthesias may radiate proximally into the distal lower leg.

Physical Examination

The classic finding is reproduction of symptoms while tapping over the tunnel (Tinel test). In severe cases, atrophy of the intrinsic muscles may be observed. Numbness may be detected over the medial and posterior calcaneus and/or arch of the foot. While observing the patient's gait, hyperpronation may be present.

Diagnostic Studies

Radiographs should be obtained to rule out bony abnormalities. An MRI is helpful to determine a structural cause of the symptoms. Ultrasound can also be used for this purpose.

Electromyelography/nerve conduction velocity studies are helpful to confirm the diagnosis and rule out other potential pathologies.

Treatment

If the patient is hyperpronating, an orthotic is helpful to correct this problem. A steroid and anesthetic injection into the tunnel (preferably done under ultrasound guidance to ensure accurate placement and avoidance of injecting the nerve or tendon) can be effective.

When aggressive conservative care does not adequately eliminate the symptoms, surgical decompression may be necessary. If a structural lesion is identified, it can be removed. If adhesions are observed on the nerve, this may be contributing to its entrapment, in which case external neurolysis may be helpful. If no structural lesion is identified on imaging, however, surgery is not as likely to be successful.

HALLUX RIGIDUS

Background

Hallux rigidus, which translates to "stiff great toe," refers to osteoarthritis (OA) of the first metatarsal phalangeal (MTP) joint. It is believed to be primarily a disease of overuse from repetitive wear and tear and hyperextension. It is most common in patients 30 to 60 years of age but may occur as early as adolescence.

Clinical Presentation

Patients generally present with complaints of pain and stiffness in their great toe. Running and other weightbearing activities tend to exacerbate the pain. Patients may note that toe-off during gait is particularly painful. If the symptoms have been present for an extended period of time, altered biomechanics may have led the patient to develop pain in the lateral aspect of the foot and/or knee. Tight shoes also exacerbate the pain.

Physical Examination

The classic examination finding is tenderness over the first MTP and increased pain with resisted dorsiflexion of the joint. An osteophyte may be palpable and tender on the dorsal aspect of the joint.

The gait may be antalgic, with the patient favoring the unaffected side and limiting the amount of toe-off because of pain and stiffness in the MTP.

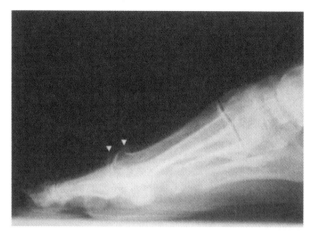

Figure 8.3 Clinical and radiographic appearance of hallux rigidus. (From Moskowitz et al. *Osteoarthritis Diagnosis and Medical/ Surgical Management*. 4th ed. Philadelphia, Pa: Lippincott Williams & Wilkins, 2007, with permission.)

Diagnostic Studies

Radiographs should be obtained and typically reveal characteristic OA findings, including joint space narrowing, spurring, osteophytes, and/or cyst formation (Fig. 8.3).

Treatment

Changing footwear to shoes with a wide toe box is helpful. A rocker bottom shoe also limits dorsiflexion of the first MTP and limits pain.

RICE is appropriate for an acute flare-up of pain. An intra-articular steroid and anesthetic injection can also help symptoms.

Multiple surgical options exist for recalcitrant symptoms. These include excision of a dorsal osteophyte, joint fusion, and osteotomy. Studies are ongoing investigating the possibility of total joint arthroplasty. It is not routinely recommended but may become more common in the future.

HALLUX VALGUS (BUNION)

Background

Hallux valgus refers to a medially deviated first metatarsal and laterally deviated first MTP joint. The medial deviation results in a prominence over the first metatarsal head, known as a bunion. The prominence can become painful. The most common cause of hallux valgus is ill-fitting shoes. Women who wear tight high-heeled shoes are particularly vulnerable to developing this condition.

Clinical Presentation

Patients complain of a prominence over their first metatarsal head that is often painful and aggravated by wearing certain shoes. Typically, the pain is relieved by taking off the offending shoes. Occasionally, patients may complain of concomitant burning, tingling, and/or numbness over the dorsal aspect of the prominence, which may reflect irritation of the medial dorsal cutaneous nerve.

Physical Examination

A prominence is noted on examination over the first metatarsal head. The first metatarsal is medially deviated and the MTP is laterally deviated. The prominence is often tender. Range of motion may be restricted.

Inspect the skin and other toes for associated deformity. The toe should also be examined in the weightbearing position.

Diagnostic Studies

Radiographs should be obtained in weightbearing and nonweightbearing to assess for degree of angulation as well as any associated bony abnormalities, including potential bony pathology in adjacent toes.

Treatment

Shoes with wide and deep toe boxes are very helpful. An orthotist may custom fit an orthotic. Tight-fitting shoes, and high heels in particular, should be avoided.

Surgical treatments include osteotomy and resectional arthroplasty, as well as others. The decision for surgical intervention, and which surgery to employ, depends on patient symptoms, degree of deformity, comorbidities, risks, and patient expectations.

Asymptomatic hallux rigidus does not require treatment, although patients should be educated about switching to different footwear if needed.

PLANTAR FASCIITIS

Background

The plantar fascia is a dense fibrous band of tissue that extends from the medial tuberosity of the calcaneus to the proximal phalanges and provides support to the foot. Plantar fasciitis is the most common cause of heel pain and believed to result from overuse, tightness of the fascia, and/or an osteophyte on the calcaneus. Of note, heel osteophytes may occur asymptomatically and do not necessarily result in symptoms. Recent weight gain (e.g., pregnancy) that increases the load of the fascia may also result in plantar fasciitis.

Clinical Presentation

Patients complain of pain primarily over the medial heel. The pain may extend along the arch of the foot. Pain is often worst in the morning with the first step of the day. This is because the plantar fascia constricts during nighttime while sleeping. Then, when the patient takes his or her first step, the plantar fascia is stretched, irritating this already inflamed and painful area. Similarly, after sitting for a prolonged period of time, getting up and putting weight on the affected foot may be painful. Walking for long distances also may exacerbate symptoms. Sitting or lying down typically alleviates the pain.

Physical Examination

The hallmark physical examination finding is point tenderness over the medial calcaneal tuberosity that reproduces the patient's symptoms. Passive dorsiflexion also may be painful. Tenderness over the lateral calcaneus should raise suspicion for a possible stress fracture.

Diagnostic Studies

None are routinely indicated. If a stress fracture is suspected, weightbearing radiographs should be obtained.

Treatment

Conservative care is very effective for plantar fasciitis. The cornerstone of treatment is ice and stretching of the plantar fascia and Achilles tendon. A formal physical therapy program may be helpful to teach the exercises. Patients should stretch their plantar fascia (using a towel to put the ankle in dorsiflexion) prior to getting up in the morning and also before putting weight on their foot after prolonged sitting during the day. A night splint to hold the ankle in dorsiflexion may also be helpful to stretch the fascia. Foot orthotics may also be helpful.

Without an injection, conservative care may take 6 to 12 months. An injection may help speed recovery, but injections in this area also carry potentially significant risks.

In patients with recalcitrant or particularly severe symptoms, an injection of anesthetic and steroid into the point of maximal tenderness on the medial calcaneus may be performed. With this injection there is a risk of heel fat pad necrosis and/or plantar fascia rupture. Using ultrasound guidance for the injection may be helpful for optimal needle placement.

Recently, some physicians have used botulinum toxin injection to treat plantar fasciitis. Initial results are promising, especially because they seem to carry fewer risks than a steroid injection. However, the cost of the toxin may be prohibitive, and more research is needed to evaluate long-term efficacy and potential side effects.

Surgery is needed in <5% of cases. Surgical options include partial plantar fascia release.

INTERDIGITAL NEUROMA (MORTON NEUROMA)

Background

An interdigital neuroma typically occurs between the third and fourth digits and less frequently occurs between the second and third digits. It rarely occurs in the first or fourth web spaces. An interdigital neuroma is a misnomer because no "neuroma" actually exists. It is in fact a compression of the interdigital nerve beneath the intermetatarsal ligament, resulting in repetitive irritation and fibrosis. A narrow toe box predisposes to this pathology. It is more common in women.

Clinical Presentation

Patients complain of pain and possibly paresthesias in the toes adjacent to the neuroma. The pain is characteristically described as "sharp" and "burning." Numbness and tingling may also be present. Wearing narrow shoes exacerbates the symptoms. Patients may report that they feel as though they are "walking on a marble." Patients typically state that sitting, removing their shoe, and rubbing their foot alleviates the symptoms.

Physical Examination

The characteristic examination finding is pain with a "squeeze test." In this test, the physician applies direct

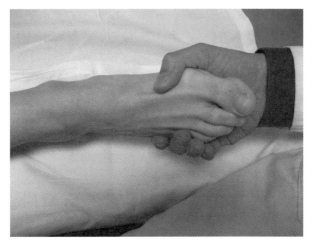

Figure 8.4   Squeeze test.

pressure to the dorsal and plantar interspace with one hand and firmly squeezes the metatarsal heads together with the other hand (Fig. 8.4). The test is considered positive for an interdigital neuroma if it reproduces symptoms.

Diagnostic Studies

None are routinely indicated.

Treatment

Wearing shoes with a low heel and wide toe box often alleviates symptoms. A metatarsal pad may also be helpful to use. An injection of steroid and anesthetic into the neuroma often provides more immediate symptom relief. Ultrasound guidance may be helpful for this injection. If one injection does not provide symptom relief, a second injection should not be performed. If conservative care is not successful, surgical excision of the neuroma may be required. An adverse reaction to surgery may be persistent dysesthesias.

METATARSALGIA

Background

The metatarsals are the long bones of the foot. The metatarsals form the part of the foot known as the "ball of the foot." Metatarsalgia refers to pain in this region. There can be multiple causes of metatarsalgia, including abnormal biomechanics. Overuse in the setting of suboptimal footwear is another common cause.

Clinical Presentation

Patients complain of pain over the plantar aspect of their forefoot over one or more of their metatarsal heads. The pain typically occurs gradually. Weightbearing and walking, in particular, may be painful.

Physical Examination

A callus may be seen over the metatarsal heads. A characteristic finding is tenderness over the plantar aspect of the metatarsal heads and fat pad. Misalignment may be present in one or more of the toes.

Diagnostic Studies

Radiographs should be obtained to rule out other bony pathology.

Treatment

A metatarsal pad is the treatment of choice for most patients. The metatarsal pad sits directly behind the painful metatarsal head. A custom-made orthotic can also be used. This treatment is generally effective. Ice can also be used in the acutely painful period. Rarely, patients continue to have pain and may require consideration of surgical toe realignment.

TURF TOE

Background

Turf toe is a hyperdorsiflexion injury of the first metatarsophalangeal (MTP) joint that is most commonly seen on artificial turf. Injury usually occurs to the capsular portion of the first MTP joint. Poor footwear that does not adequately support the foot during athletic competition or training may also predispose to turf toe.

Clinical Presentation

Patients complain of pain, stiffness, and swelling over their first MTP. The injury often begins after an acute injury but may result from repetitive strain. Typically, patients report having participated in an athletic event (e.g., football) on artificial turf. Following the injury, walking, running, cutting, and pivoting on the affected foot may be difficult. Patients may also report having inexpensive athletic footwear.

Physical Examination

The classic examination finding is pain with end range dorsiflexion of the first MTP. The first MTP is also typically tender, stiff, and often swollen. Ecchymosis may also be present.

Diagnostic Studies

Radiographs may be obtained to rule out bony abnormality.

Gout may appear similar to turf toe clinically. If there is no acute injury, or if the patient has not recently competed in an athletic event on artificial turf (or if the patient has a history of gout), gout should be suspected and the joint should be aspirated.

Treatment

PRICE should be performed in the acutely painful period. Taping the toe in a plantar-flexed position may also be helpful. The patient should wear only footwear that supports the foot adequately. A rocker bottom sole or stiff-soled shoe is appropriate. Rigid turf-toe orthotics may be helpful. Surgical intervention is generally not necessary unless radiographs reveal an associated fracture (e.g., avulsion fracture).

ACHILLES TENDON RUPTURE

Background

Achilles tendon rupture typically occurs in active, healthy adults from 30 to 50 years of age who participate in weekend sports. The rupture occurs approximately 1 to 2 inches proximal to the tendon's insertion on the calcaneus.

Clinical Presentation

Patients present with an acute episode of severe calf pain that feels as if they were "shot" or "kicked very hard" in their calf. They may report feeling a "snap" or "pop" in their calf. The severe pain resolves and the patient is left with calf swelling and weakness. Some patients are initially told they have a bad ankle sprain. Patients are unable to stand on their toes on the affected side. Stair climbing is difficult, and the patient often complains of an altered gait.

In some patients, a history of heel pain and/or Achilles tendon pain may be present. This may suggest an acute injury in the setting of a weakened fibrotic tendon. However, in many patients, there is no history of heel or tendon pain.

Less often, patients may report actually being struck in the Achilles tendon by a kick or other trauma that precipitated symptoms.

Physical Examination

A palpable defect is detected along the tendon in a full rupture. Swelling is typically present. The patient is unable to toe-stand on the affected limb. The classic test is the Thompson test (Figs. 8.5A and B). In this test, the patient lies prone with the affected leg extended so that the knee

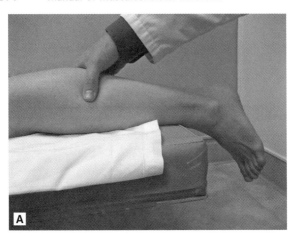

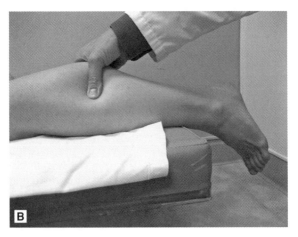

Figure 8.5   Thompson test.

is supported on the examining table but the lower leg
hangs off it. The physician then squeezes the calf muscles.
In a normal functioning limb, the foot should respond by
plantarflexing. However, if a rupture is present, the foot
does not plantarflex.

Diagnostic Studies

None are routinely ordered. Radiographs may be obtained to rule out associated bony abnormality. Ultrasound or MRI may be obtained to confirm the diagnosis if in doubt, particularly if a partial rupture is suspected.

Treatment

Conservative care includes a progressive casting immobilization program in which the ankle is initially casted in mild plantarflexion and then gradually moved to the neutral position. This is followed by a physical therapy program that focuses on gentle stretching and strengthening.

Surgical care reattaches the tendon and may be done percutaneously or through an open approach. Following surgery, patients are placed in a cast or walking boot for approximately 6 to 12 weeks. As with conservative care, the foot is typically placed initially in mild plantarflexion and then may be gradually moved to the neutral position with serial bracing. After casting, patients begin a physical therapy program.

Conservative care has a higher incidence of re-rupture in patients. However, conservative care does not have the inherent risks of surgery. In general, surgery may be more appropriate in younger, active patients who wish to return to competitive sports. All the benefits and risks of surgical versus conservative intervention (given the patient's comorbidities, level of activity, etc.) should be discussed with the patient. Importantly, treatment should be instituted as soon as possible to help prevent further morbidity.

MEDIAL CALF INJURY (TENNIS LEG)

Background

A medial calf injury, or tear, has been called "tennis leg" because of its propensity to occur during tennis. However, as with "tennis elbow," this injury can occur in a variety of sports and activities. It is most common in the "weekend warrior" athlete who is not properly conditioned but then exerts himself or herself on the weekend. Typically, the injury occurs during "push-off" from a position in which the knee is extended and the ankle dorsiflexed.

Clinical Presentation

Patients typically report a "popping" or "tearing" sensation occurred in their calf while pushing off their foot. Common complaints include pain and swelling, predominantly in the medial calf.

Physical Examination

The medial calf is typically tender and swelling is noted. Importantly, the Achilles tendon should be palpated and found to be intact. The Thompson test (in which the calf is squeezed and the foot plantarflexes if the Achilles tendon is intact) is negative. Ankle range of motion is often restricted secondary to pain. Dorsiflexion increases the pain.

Diagnostic Studies

Radiographs are not always ordered but may be obtained to rule out an avulsion fracture. Ultrasound or MRI are not routinely indicated unless the diagnosis is in doubt. Ultrasound is appropriate if the presentation is atypical and/or a deep venous thrombosis is suspected.

Treatment

PRICE is the cornerstone of treatment. Physical therapy that focuses on stretching and strengthening is an important part of treatment. The patient should also be instructed to continue a home exercise program and appropriate warm-up exercises prior to sports in the future to reduce the risk of recurrent injury.

MEDIAL TIBIAL STRESS SYNDROME (SHIN SPLINTS)

Background

Medial tibial stress syndrome is known as "shin splints" because it results in pain along the anterior tibia. Shin splints are an overuse injury common in runners and sports that require a lot of running. Poor footwear, running on an uneven surface, and running down hills are often contributory factors. Recent increase in level of activity also may predispose to developing shin splints. If shin splints are not addressed early, a tibial stress fracture may develop.

Clinical Presentation

Patients initially complain of pain over their shin when running. If not addressed, the symptoms progress so the pain becomes more frequent and ultimately may become constant. Patients do not generally note significant swelling.

Physical Examination

Tenderness is typically present over the medial tibia. Swelling, if present, is generally minimal.

Diagnostic Studies

This is generally a clinical diagnosis. However, if a stress fracture is suspected, radiographs and/or a bone scan may be needed.

Treatment

PRICE is the cornerstone of treatment. If the patient hyperpronates or has low arches, an arch support or custom orthotic may be very helpful. It is also important to make sure that the patient is wearing appropriate footwear. Activities should be modified to be pain free.

Physical therapy may be helpful to stretch and strengthen the surrounding muscles and help prevent recurrence. When running is reinstituted, it must be done gradually to make sure that it does not provoke pain.

ANTERIOR ANKLE IMPINGEMENT

Background

Anterior ankle impingement is an irritation and inflammation of the joint capsule and surrounding ligaments and soft tissues. The most common cause is posttraumatic, such as after a severe ankle sprain or multiple ankle sprains. However, it also may occur as a repetitive use injury such as in athletes (e.g., baseball catchers) and dancers that require repetitive dorsiflexion. If an osteophyte has developed as a result of overuse, this may impinge the soft tissues during repetitive dorsiflexion.

Clinical Presentation

Patients typically complain of achy anterior and anterolateral ankle pain that is exacerbated by participation in dance or sport. Patients may report a history of an ankle sprain or other ankle injury in the past. Patients may report that their ankle feels somewhat "unsteady."

Physical Examination

Tenderness to palpation is noted over the perceived painful area. Minimal swelling may be present. Range of motion of the ankle may be slightly restricted secondary to pain. Passive dorsiflexion may reproduce pain. Having the patient perform a squat typically reproduces symptoms.

Diagnostic Studies

Radiographs may be helpful. MRI may also be helpful, although it has a low sensitivity for picking up lesions in this condition. MRI is useful to help exclude other potential pathologies.

Treatment

The cornerstone of treatment is PRICE. Physical therapy may also be helpful. If the patient is a dancer or athlete, technique should be assessed to ensure that undue stress is not being placed on the anterior ankle. Some physicians advocate an intra-articular steroid and anesthetic injection performed ideally under ultrasound guidance. Occasionally, some physicians may place their patients in a walking boot for a short period of time.

In resistant cases, surgical intervention may be necessary. Arthroscopic excision of any offending osteophyte and/or debridement of the capsule may be performed.

POSTERIOR ANKLE IMPINGEMENT

Background

In approximately 10% to 15% of the population, the lateral tuberosity of the talus does not communicate directly with the talus. When this happens, the lateral tuberosity is called an os trigonum and sits between the talus and calcaneus. Ballet dancers spend a lot of time in *en pointe* and *demi pointe* positions. These positions require plantar hyperflexion, which creates additional stress on the posterior portion of the ankle. Ballet dancers with an os trigonum are particularly vulnerable to developing posterior ankle impingement syndrome.

Of course, any athlete *can* develop posterior impingement. However, because most sports do not require repetitive plantar hyperflexion, they are less likely to lead to posterior impingement.

A history of an ankle injury may also precipitate posterior impingement, particularly in ballet dancers, if the ankle is less stable after the injury (e.g., significant sprain).

Clinical Presentation

Patients are typically ballet dancers who present with posterior heel pain or deep ankle pain that is exacerbated by *en pointe* and *demi pointe* positions.

Physical Examination

On examination, patients characteristically have tenderness over the inferior edge of the fibula. While maintaining compression over the inferior fibula and calcaneus, moving the ankle into plantar flexion exacerbates the pain.

Diagnostic Studies

Radiographs are indicated to identify the os trigonum, if present.

Treatment

As with anterior impingement, the cornerstone of treatment is PRICE. Physical therapy may also be helpful. An injection, preferably under ultrasound guidance, of steroid and anesthetic into the area between the os trigonum (if present) and talus and/or calcaneus may be helpful.

In resistant cases, surgical removal of the os trigonum or posterior lateral tubercle (if not separated) may be necessary.

FLEXOR HALLUCIS LONGUS TENDONITIS

Background

The flexor hallucis longus (FHL) tendon runs deeply through the tarsal tunnel. In athletes requiring repetitive push off, the tendon may become inflamed. Dancers who compensate for a lack of hip turnout by externally rotating their lower leg and turning out only their lower feet compress the tarsal tunnel mechanically and are at increased risk of FHL tendonitis. Patients with hyperpronation who dance or play sports also may be at slightly increased risk.

Clinical Presentation

Patients are typically dancers or athletes who present with complaints of pain in the medial malleolus and along the course of the FHL. The great toe may occasionally trigger because of tendinosis of the tendon. Symptoms are worsened during toe-off, and participation in dance (particularly during *en pointe* or *demi pointe* positions) or sports.

Physical Examination

The tendon runs deeply in the tarsal tunnel and is not typically tender in this area. Weakness may be appreciated in the first MTP during plantarflexion. Patients may have reproduction of symptoms during standing on the affected extremity and repeatedly plantarflexing that foot.

Diagnostic Studies

Radiographs may be obtained to rule out bony pathology. Ultrasound and/or MRI may also be helpful to confirm the diagnosis and help rule out other pathologies such as a torn tendon.

Treatment

Conservative care includes activity modification and PRICE. If patients participate in dance or other sporting activity, their technique should be evaluated and possibly modified to be biomechanically optimal. If the patient hyperpronates or has a flat foot, an orthotic may be helpful. Some patients may benefit from an injection of steroid and anesthetic in the tarsal tunnel (ideally performed under ultrasound guidance).

If symptoms persist despite aggressive conservative care, surgical debridement may be required.

ANKLE AND FOOT STRESS FRACTURES

Background

As in other parts of the body, a stress fracture in the lower leg, ankle, or foot is an overuse injury. Stress fractures can occur at multiple points in the lower leg, ankle, and foot. The most common location in the foot is the second metatarsal followed by the third metatarsal (these are sometimes called "march fractures" because military recruits marching often suffer this injury). Athletes, dancers, and military recruits are at particular risk. A sudden increase in level of activity or change in surface on which activity is performed, precipitating the gradual onset of painful symptoms, should prompt suspicion for stress fracture.

A stress fracture in a young woman should prompt clinical suspicion for the female athlete triad. A stress fracture in an older man or woman should prompt clinical suspicion for osteoporosis.

Clinical Presentation

Patients typically report gradual onset of pain in the setting of recently increasing activity or changing the surface on which they were training. For example, a military recruit accustomed to a predominantly sedentary lifestyle is at particular risk for a stress fracture during basic training. A runner who moves to running on the streets of his town after running on an indoor track all winter is also at increased risk.

There may be diffuse swelling in addition to pain.

Physical Examination

Tenderness is appreciated over the fracture. Swelling and ecchymosis may also be present.

Diagnostic Studies

Radiographs may not reveal the fracture until 4 weeks after the onset of symptoms. Bone scan is typically positive

1 to 3 days after symptom onset, although it may take up to 5 days for this test to be positive as well.

MRI is largely becoming the modality of choice for diagnosing stress fractures in the foot and ankle. MRI has a higher specificity than bone scan and can be positive 24 hours after symptom onset.

Treatment

Patients with a metatarsal stress fracture can be treated conservatively with PRICE and immobilization in a wooden-soled shoe or short CAM Walker.

If the stress fracture is in the fifth metatarsal, however, there is a higher risk of nonunion. These patients require closer observation and possible earlier surgical intervention with screw and possible bone graft (depending on the patient's desire to return to activity sooner).

Conservative treatment for a fifth metatarsal stress fracture includes being immobilized in a short leg cast for 6 to 8 weeks. If a nonunion develops, surgical intervention with screw fixation is needed.

Patients with navicular and talus stress fractures have a high rate of nonunion and require immobilization and possible earlier surgical intervention.

Calcaneus and fibula stress fractures tend to respond well to PRICE and immobilization.

If a patient is suspected of having the female athlete triad (disordered eating, amenorrhea, and osteoporosis), she should receive appropriate education, counseling, and follow-up care. Likewise, if the patient is older and suspected of having osteoporosis, appropriate care must be initiated.

Index

Page numbers followed by *f*, *t*, or *b* denote figure, table, or box, respectively.